I0767057

DIARY OF A MAD PRACTITIONER

THE ANGRY PANCREAS AND OTHER TALES OF EFT TAPPING

DR. ROSSANNA M. MASSEY

To George, Dad, Mom, Louie, and Coco, with all my love and gratitude.

And the day came when the risk to remain tight in a bud was more painful than the risk it took to blossom.

– Author: Anaïs Nin

Can you remember who you were before the world told you who you should be?

– Author: Unknown

To Thine Own Self Be True

– Author: William Shakespeare

An arrow can only be shot by pulling it backward. When you feel like you are being dragged back by difficulties, it means you are torquing up to launch forward. Stay focused and keep aiming.

– Author: Unknown

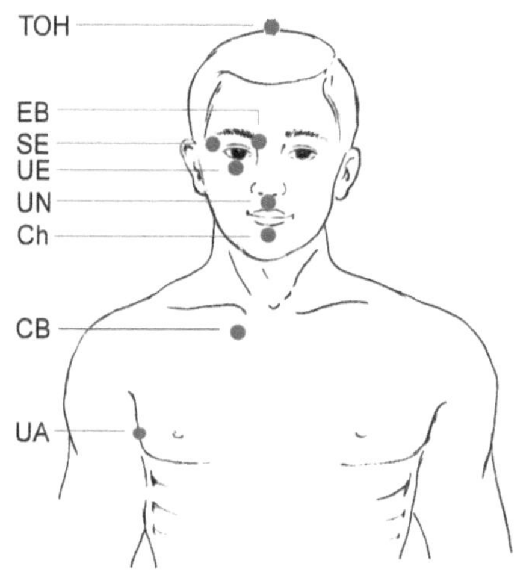
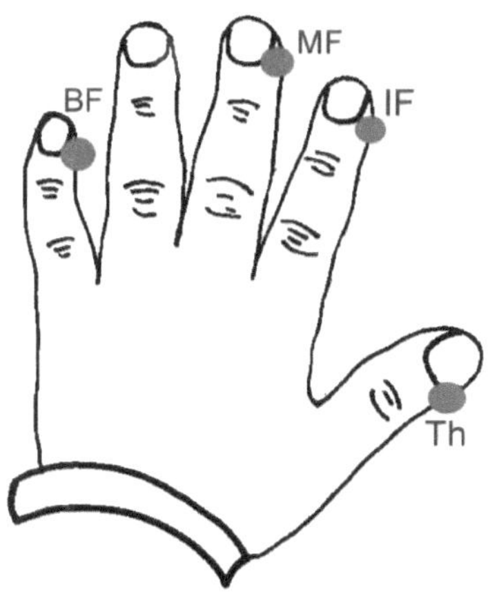

TOH - top of head   UA - under arm
EB - eyebrow   Th - thumb
SE - side of eye   IF - index finger
UE - under eye   MF - middle finger
UN - under nose   BF - baby finger
Ch - chin

New to Emotional Freedom Techniques? Please reference chapter 5, EFT Cliff Notes and Appendix I for a brief orientation to the procedures used in EFT 'tapping.'

CONTENTS

PART IV

PART V

PART VI

PART VII

APPENDICES

I f you're new to the subject of what has come to be called "Tapping", then this book is a must.

If you've known about tapping and EFT for quite some time, then this book is a must.

"Diary" is fairly loosely used as a way to help conceptualize Dr. Rossanna's journey from childhood to internationally known EFT Practitioner. She weaves the stories that make up her life into a captivating and insightful backdrop for her patient's and client's EFT experiences.

Early on in her exploration of EFT, she had no interest in focusing on serious diseases and pain syndromes, even though she was a chiropractic physician. Her real interest was in personal development and confidence building, but the serious diseases would not leave her be. So, gradually she resigned herself to the fact that people with serious conditions needed her because they just kept coming. It turns out, her life's work was hidden in her resistance.

Perhaps it was her clinical background and perspective or maybe it was her strong, intuitive insights into the emotional layers of the person she was talking to. Whatever the blending of skills, she proved to be remarkably effective with her clients.

It was apparently because so many of her clients were in dire straits health-wise, even terminal stage 4 cancers, that Dr. Rossanna's approach evolved into a "No Pussy-footing Around", "Cut to the Quick", and "Go for the Jugular" way of speeding things along. Time was of the essence. Out of that slowly developed what has become her Bitch Tap Method™.

It wasn't an easy evolution. As a professional, it's not at all accepted protocol to use cussing and even vulgarity with a patient or client. And many resisted moving into more forceful and angry language, feeling that it was somehow "un-evolved", "immoral" or "unspiritual."

And yet, the breakthroughs she got with her sessions, the deep purges of choked off anger and resentment, whenever she got full-on participation in her approach were stunning.

I said at the beginning that this book is a 'must'. I say that because it will restore your enthusiasm for using EFT on yourself if you're an old hand and it will inspire you with a vision of the many ways your life can benefit knowing "tapping" if you're a newbie.

This is not a book about how to learn EFT. There are many wonderful programs, workshops and books that will help you do that. This is a book about the human side of being a practitioner, about how your own past experiences shape who you've become and how EFT can remove blinders and filters that prevent you from being healthier, being better, being more.

George A. Massey, D.C.

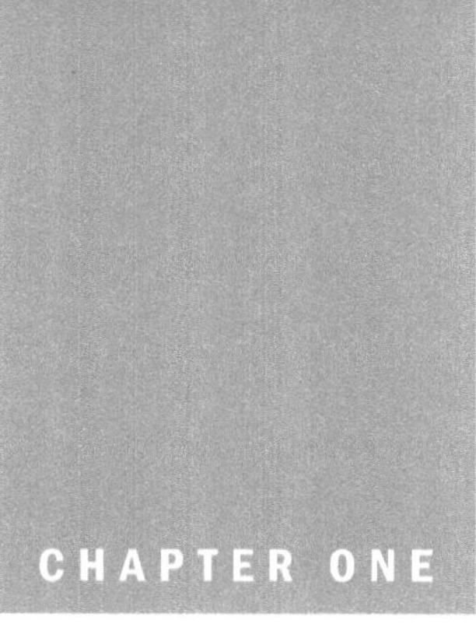

The Angry Pancreas

**The doctor says,"You have pancreatic cancer.
You have 6 months to live, a year at most."**

What do you do now?

With that my EFT career started off with a BANG! Knowing that the survival rate for pancreatic cancer was low, I knew it wasn't going to turn out well. I took this case on anyway. Because I've always been fearless, and because "Karen" was a pseudonym for a beloved aunt of mine.

Spontaneous healing from a cancerous pancreatic tumor as it turns out is a very big deal. I sat there dazed in front of my computer stunned by the thousands of emails from people across the globe. Those emails for help came in a constant flow every day for weeks, and months afterward. I never expected so much attention from all over the world: Egypt, Israel, Africa, Dubai, India, South America, Germany, Japan, Sweden, the UK, Australia, New Zealand, Tobago, everywhere. I was officially global.

I'm not exaggerating when I say that I woke up to thousands of emails from all over the world after I'd submitted my article. It was highlighted as the top story on the home page Emofree.com, Gary Craig's EFT global website. The story was an overnight sensation, placing me smack-dab in the middle of the "EFT" spotlight.

My aunt and I were to be featured in an upcoming movie about EFT. My career as a practitioner was about to blow up exponentially! Oh, the thrill of it all, it was unbelievable! It was such an exhilarating time for me, and I'm grateful for being able to experience that type of career head-rush. It was amazing.

For the record, I'd like to reinforce my insider's guide to our sessions. I let go of the outcome, no healing agenda whatsoever. The doctor part of me knew it was almost impossible to stop pancreatic cancer. Everyone knows it's a death sentence, nobody survives it. So I tapped for letting go of that limited belief (nobody survives it) before our initial session. I left our sessions open-ended and approached the treatments as strictly palliative. My intention was not to cure but to merely help her drop the negative emotions trapped in her energy system. Period. The results were astounding.

"The Angry Pancreas." as published on EMOFREE.com.

Since the beginning of my EFT career, I've been fascinated by the many layers of emotion behind serious diseases. Many of my patients who came to me for spinal related problems were also under their medical doctor's care for a variety of different illnesses. Intuitively I always suspected specific emotions related to their chronic illnesses, yet I was careful not to approach the subject with them. My patients would tell you that I am not a shy person, but I was mindful not to get too personal while working on them. I did notice, however, the "trends" of emotions that went along with their particular illnesses. In the many thousands of patients I've seen in my seventeen-year career as a Chiropractor, I've yet to meet a cancer patient who wasn't angry.

Here is a cancer story that not is only miraculous, but a real testimony of how EFT heals people on a cellular, energetic level. Before I begin, I'd like to add that since this experience, I now cringe when I hear other people describe their "battle" with cancer or their "fight" with it. Why not approach cancer by waving the white flag, honoring what your body is trying to tell you, and make peace with it?

A year ago I found out that a dear friend of mine, Karen, who lives in Texas was diagnosed with pancreatic cancer, and had a bleak prognosis. She had been seeking alternative methods of treatment because the consequences of the medical "slash and burn" techniques were in her opinion, unacceptable. She knew I had been studying EFT as an advanced practitioner. Karen wanted to leave nothing out of her holistic regimen, so gave me a call and asked for my help. Finally, I thought, this was my first experience with treating the emotions behind cancer, and I jumped at the opportunity. We arranged our weekly phone sessions, and I advised her to come up with her own "personal peace" list.

Gary, I must admit that in the back of my mind I was insecure about the outcome of our sessions, and of disappointing her as well. So I tapped on myself accordingly; "Even though I'm afraid she'll die anyway because this is incurable, I deeply love and respect myself." "Even though I feel guilty that she trusts me to help her, and I may fail, I deeply love and accept myself" "Even though I have no business dealing with this serious illness, I choose to be calm and relaxed about it," "Even though she may be too far gone, at the very least, she can die in peace." And most importantly to me, "Even though I need to save her, I love myself, and understand where this is coming from." Once I got myself sufficiently out of the way, I was ready for our first phone session.

I was not surprised by the short length of her personal peace list. She was always one to "gloss over" painful events and pretend things didn't bother her. By choosing not to engage in confrontations, or defend herself over the years with her critical in-laws, she ended up stuffing down large amounts of anger that even she was surprised she still had, in spite of her passive "adult" way of handling things. I've always thought that anger is such a difficult emotion to deal with due to the very thick shell of denial that is wrapped around it. Since I already knew most of her issues through the years, I decided not to approach any of them directly, and instead get right to the sick pancreas to ask it for its painful priority. Her medical doctor told her that her CAT scan showed she had a large mass at the head of her pancreas consistent with malignancy, and that it was putting pressure on her surrounding organs making her jaundiced. She had lost a lot of weight and had no appetite.

The first corridor to go through was her lack of self-acceptance. I like to have my clients first say aloud "I deeply and profoundly love and accept myself." I ask how it feels intellectually, and I get one answer, then ask I how they feel emotionally and get quite another. After three rounds of "Even though I can't love or accept myself, I choose to try," I moved to the next barrier and asked her what she imagined her sick pancreas looked like. What color is it? She replied, "It's definitely black." Then I asked her what texture it was, and she described it as lumpy. What would it smell like? And she said, "foul, like something died." If it had an emotion, what would it be? "It would be angry." Because Karen was so dissociated with her anger, we began with the long version of the tapping sequence to leave no stone unturned. "Even though I have anger in my 'head', and there's so much of it, I don't know where to begin, I deeply love myself." The first round of tapping was enough to shake loose her first subconscious priority of painful memories. "My mother in law never liked me, and let me know how disappointed she was that my husband didn't marry his ex-girlfriend Sandra instead."

Gary, I want everyone to know that this healing experience didn't happen overnight. It took one and a half months which, in itself, is still amazing. Adding to the urgency of the situation was that her husband and daughters were pressuring her into returning to the medical doctors for another CAT scan, and schedule the proposed surgery to remove her pancreas, (slash) and have chemo with radiation (burn.) Working against the clock, we stepped up our sessions to twice weekly.

Since I didn't have the luxury of time to step politely around her issues, I developed my own "Massey Emotional Trigger Point Technique" (my Bitch Tap Method™ precursor). This directly addresses the abject negativity of her thoughts and is "pressed" on it until it's cleared (this is similar to the deep tissue-work technique which is quite painful but very effective in releasing "trapped" physical tensions). I also encouraged her to use "spicy" language to step up her pancreatic purge. Our set-up phrases were as follows:

"Even though I was taught to show respect for my elders, I still hate Mrs. Dexter, and I refuse to forgive her." Reminder phrase; "I hate her g.d. guts, I refuse to forgive her!"

Even though her mother in law was now deceased, I knew it would be a good idea for Karen to finally tell her off, out loud, instead of doing it in her "head." Here's how that went; "Even though I didn't have the courage to tell you then, I deeply love and accept myself, and you're a vicious and jealous old hag, and I can't stand you either! At each tapping point, I had her plug in all the things she could never say, and even yell it out!

She was exhausted after that round of tapping but said she felt warm and relaxed. We resumed our next session later on in the week.

"Even though I wasn't good enough to please her."

"Even though I could never hurt my husband by saying it, your mama is a B*!*#!"

Reminder phrase was; "She's a B*!*#!" She's such a damn B*!*#!"

"Even though his whole family thinks he could have done better."

"Even though it matters to me what they think."

"Even though I'm stupid for letting their opinions get to me."

"Even though he's stupid for taking all their abuse."

"Even though I hate myself for staying with him for so long and putting up with this s*!t."

"Even though I'm pissed at him for not defending me against his mother."

"Even though my daughters got snubbed by them when they were little and innocent."

The first week after our initial session Karen reported that her appetite was returning and that she felt more peaceful. In two weeks, she was no longer jaundiced. With every week that passed, she started to feel more comfortable and started recognizing her issues about her own parents without feeling like she was dishonoring them. As in the case of most angry people, she felt that she had already "dealt" with that part of her life, but I knew better. She admitted that her mother was bossy and controlling who "picked on" her father, who never defended himself. The guilt behind the anger at her own parents, who are both deceased, kept her from ever expressing it. I assured her that you can love someone very deeply and still be angry at them. It is about finding clarity, and forgiveness of one's self, and of them.

What happened at our last session the day before her CAT scan was truly amazing, and it still gives me chills whenever I think about it. All the while I worked on Karen I knew the culmination of our work together was to be the issue of forgiveness. So we began;

"Even though I put my anger in the head of my pancreas, so I could clear my own head, I deeply and profoundly love and accept myself, and I honor my pancreas for working so hard to protect me."

Reminder phrase; "Gratitude for my pancreas, and all that it's done for me, it's safe to let go now."

"Even though I've held a grudge for his family for so long now it's killing me, I deeply love and accept myself, and for my own sake I want to release it." Reminder phrases; "They could never feel my anger only I did now I'm paying for it," "I only hurt myself."

We hadn't even finished the tapping sequence when Karen said, "I feel sorry for Mrs. Dexter, she was critical of me because maybe she didn't like herself. It must have made her feel better to find fault with me. I'm sure she was critical of her own children too. Maybe that's why they listened to her and went along with it. What child doesn't want their parent's approval?"

My last set-up phrase was the key that unlocked the door to her pancreatic head, and allowed the release of its anger in a most unexpected way;

"In spite of all the years they caused me anguish and pain, on a cellular level, I forgive them all with every fiber of my being." Reminder phrase; I forgive them with every fiber of my being, I forgive them on a deep cellular level, I forgive them with all my heart and soul, it feels wonderful to feel true forgiveness and really mean it."

Karen stopped tapping and declared she felt a very sharp pain in the left upper quadrant of her abdomen. And then said; "This is embarrassing but I just passed the most horrible gas that is so foul smelling, it's like something died inside of me! I never in my life had gas like this before, and it's so bad I have to leave the room! I told her to call me back after the "smoke cleared," and waited for her call.

Karen called back about ten minutes later to tell me she had to ventilate the room before entering it so she could call me back. She said, "My whole body feels like it's tingling, and I'm so relaxed." I asked her to close her eyes and describe what color her pancreas was, and she said that it was pink and shiny. When asked about the texture, she proclaimed that it was smooth. If she could smell it, how would it smell? She replied, "Just like fresh air."

If it had an emotion, what would it be? "It's happy, and the face on the head is smiling, and so am I!"

We ended our call with her thanking me profusely for all of my efforts, and assured me that no matter the outcome, she would forever be grateful for the EFT sessions. She promised to call me after her doctor's appointment to let me know the results of all the testing and her date of surgery.

CHAPTER TWO

The Let Down

The next day Karen called me and asked me to tap her for fear as they were driving to meet with the Oncologist and the surgeon. "Even though both of these doctors intimidate me, and have pressured me in the past about this surgery, I love and accept who I am, and I honor and trust my own inner wisdom to know what is best for me." "Even though these doctors threaten me and make me feel stupid for not listening to them, I deeply love and forgive myself for feeling stupid, and I forgive them because they're only doing what they think is right."

For fear of adding extra pressure on Karen and her family, I refrained from calling her and kept my distance hoping for the best possible outcome. Two weeks later I received a call from a mutual friend who said, "Did you hear about Karen?" My heart leaped into my throat as I asked: "No, why?" "Well, they can't find any trace of cancer in her pancreas, and whatever mass there was in the first scan, was completely gone in the second one!"

I felt elated for the outcome yet kind of sad and puzzled that she didn't tell me the good news herself. I picked up the phone and called her. She was glad to hear from me and apologized for not calling. She and her whole family, including his relatives, were celebrating her profound recovery. She told me that her blood work and CAT scan findings were all normal, and quite a contrast to the first time they were taken. Her doctors were entirely dumbfounded by their findings and said that in all the years they've treated patients, neither one of them have ever experienced a spontaneous healing. The mass at the head of her pancreas was gone entirely, and she was deemed cancer-free.

It was beginning to feel like one of the most blatant examples of the Apex Effect In EFT, the Apex Effect refers to the situation where a person has a sudden positive change but discounts EFT as being the cause until she whispered into the telephone; "I know this is all because of EFT, but my husband doesn't believe it. He thinks it's because of all the special prayers he said for me. You know how deeply religious he is. I can't thank you enough for all your help. God and EFT saved my life."

Upon a one-year follow-up appointment with her doctors, there was still not a trace of anything wrong, and she's clean as a whistle.

Emotional freedom can only bring you peace, and it's never been about the battle with cancer, it's all in the surrender.

Because of the intense interest and the response from people all over the world, Gary Craig called me. After I got over the shock of hearing his voice on the phone, it was amazing to speak to an incredible guy like Gary Craig. It was the first of many phone conversations between us planning out how this all would unfold once I had proof. There would be a movie about EFT, and our success story was to be highlighted. I arranged to meet with the movie's cinematographer in Texas to film a meeting with my aunt.

I called and asked her if she would allow the release of her records, and she said she'd think about it. I decided to travel to Texas and speak to her in person. I'd bring the release form to her, and make sure the forms were delivered to her doctors.

At about the same time, in 2008, our world in Michigan was falling apart. George and I continued to lose ground financially. Thanks to my dad, who bought two tickets to Texas, I took my mom along for support. But we were both in for a great big shock.

Although I told her that we were flying out to see her and talk about the whole thing, my aunt chose not to answer her phone. WTF? Undaunted, I had to use the precious little time I had available to uncover the real truth. Did it really happen? How could that be a lie? But I had never been treated in this manner before by any relative. I felt sad.

I was embarrassed, and my feelings were hurt for being treated like someone she felt she had to run away from. In what I can only describe as disbelief, I actually drove to their house, twice. While their cars were there, they refused to answer the door.

I had brought along a medical record release form to be signed by her and submitted to her oncologist and surgeons. That would never happen.

Finally, on our last night there before my mom and I flew home, they showed up where we were staying purely as a gesture of acknowledgment that mom was in town. They acted estranged, not at all warm and familiar. My aunt made it clear she was not on board to be in a movie about her recovery, she did not want anyone to know anything about her. It just wasn't in her nature to have that type of attention. I offered to have her face blurred on camera (as suggested by the cinematographer) but her answer was still no. My uncle flat-out told me that nothing I did helped, this stupid tapping thing was a joke, it doesn't work, and that his prayers to God were what healed her, not me. I didn't think I healed her either, I was just the facilitator. It was the EFT that purged all that negative emotional garbage out of her tissues.

I don't deny that the will of God is instrumental in all healing. God gives us the knowledge to find the right tools for us to play an active role in our recovery. That is why people seek doctors and healers to assist in the process.

But there it was. If I tried any harder for evidence, I would have been a stalker. The thrill of appearing in a movie about EFT, the possibilities for my career and being able to stay afloat while our house and clinic sold...all vanished. I decided the healthiest thing for me was not to pursue it any further, for my own sake I had to let it go and walk away. I would never be able to find out the truth, I had to be cool with that.

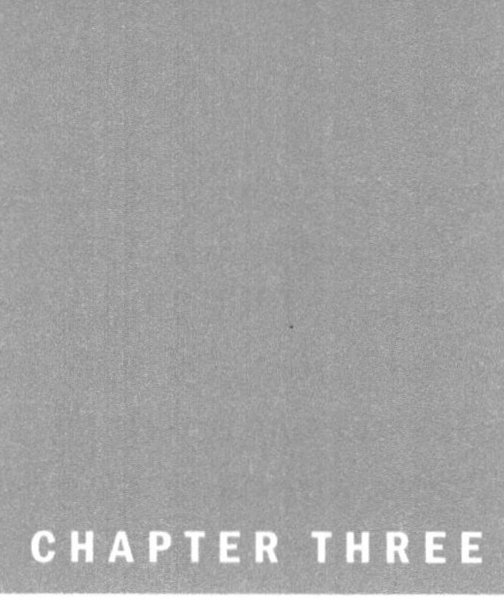

CHAPTER THREE

Onward And Upward

I came home completely defeated, bitterly disappointed, and totally humiliated. I dreaded making that phone call to Gary. It was so tough for me to have to explain that my own aunt, who accepted my help, was not going to help me in return, or anyone else for that matter. Gary was very kind, but I knew he was deeply disappointed, I could hear it in his voice. I felt like a complete and utter fool because now, Gary must think my family is composed of total flakes. As embarrassed as I was to speak to him after everything we'd been through, I could tell that he felt my sincerity, he still had faith in me.

Left to make up my own ending to the story, I chose one that made the most sense based on our past conversations. For Karen's own reasons, it was a way to make my uncle pay attention to her, and show how much he cared. My final conclusion could only be that she had to have lied.

I want you all to know that EFT is the primary tool I use for my daily emotional hygiene. If I hadn't known about EFT, I guarantee you it would have been my defeat, and I would have brooded about it for years, licked my wounds, and gone nowhere. But I used EFT to help me work through all the major buttons that were pushed. The deep humiliation, deep frustration, helplessness, anger, sadness, worthlessness, embarrassment. Who did I think I was anyway?

I got through the gigantic let-down by using EFT to snap myself out of the emotional funk it caused me. But I still had "blind spots," the residual feelings about it, the unanswered questions. It would cast me adrift career-wise for years afterward.

I considered this event to be one of the greatest loose ends of my career, one that tarnished my credibility. There was no other way.

To help expand the scope of EFT, I began to receive private client referrals from Gary, the "hard cases." If I did it once, I could do it again. Picking myself back up and dusting myself off, I put my game face on, and carried on with my work without looking back.

But the article stayed alive and kept popping up like a tap on the shoulder as if that whole sensation around the miraculous event refused to die. It would remain to be a constant reminder for many years after the fact, one that I could neither prove nor deny. Through their own research, desperately ill clients would still seek me out on the internet. My clients had faith in the process, and rightly so. I could run, but I couldn't hide.

Fast forward...George and I are now living in New Mexico, and that meant the occasional but unavoidable family gatherings. And that meant the possibility of seeing my now "healed" aunt and my uncle for the first time. Determined to relax and be myself, (like I know how to be anything else) we all met and said hello. It was a warm, familiar greeting, and as we exchanged pleasantries, I waited to see who would bring it up first, but no one ever said another word about it. Everyone's over it, and nothing ever happened. Subject closed.

Time passed, but on three separate occasions, as it turned out, each one of her sons pulled me aside privately to thank me for helping their mother. They stressed the point of how much I really helped her. They were all very loving and gracious. Their acknowledgment took me by surprise because I never expected that to happen, it never was praise I was after anyhow. I only wanted proof, and to provide hope for others.

The Backstory to The Angry Pancreas

This represents one of the most dramatic, and tumultuous times of my life. It actually took a full decade until I was able to muster up the courage and reach out to call one of her sons, (my cousin), to find out what really happened. I had nothing left to lose.

In the long run, it was their candidness and sincerity that reopened the Pandora's box of curiosity. I had questions, many questions. And, after all this time, I had to work up enough nerve to call one of her sons. I told myself (while tapping): Okay, you can't just sit on your hands and do nothing anymore, take a stand, what's wrong with you girl? Aren't you even curious to know WTF happened? Reach out and call him, do you hear me? What's the worst that could happen, you get hung up on? Get over it! Go on, call him, do it! Lol, I'm my own best cheerleader, what can I say? Doing that while tapping works every time!

We agreed upon an appointed time for us to speak by phone. It turned out to be a very relaxed, sweet and friendly conversation. After all this time, my questions were finally answered by her own son, an insider, who personally witnessed this event, and I mean all of it. This is a transcript of our recorded conversation, with his permission, because I didn't want to miss a thing he said. Here's what he said.

> "My mom talked to me about what you had done, and then she showed me some article you did. You know, it was the damnedest thing, they had so many doctors looking at her, and my mom was yellow as could be, she had every symptom that you could find for pancreatic cancer. She had everything you could think of, it was very bad. She'd lost some weight, not that she had so much to lose.
>
> The doctors did quite a few endoscopies, Cat scans, MRIs, name it all, they did it. Mom's claustrophobic, so I would go with her at the imagining place and hold her hand while they did the MRI. Through it all my mom was very positive and started opening up to me after a few weeks, maybe a month had passed. I knew she had talked with you already, before that, my brother took her down to Houston to see an Asian medicine doctor. She said; "I'm not going to let medical doctors cut me open."
>
> They could never find the actual growth, they would see it in an image, and when they ran further testing, it was gone. You know my mom, she's kinda like you, she

does the holistic approach, and believes in other things. Through it all my dad had no idea what was going on, it was a tough time, it was scary. But at the same time, I said mom, if you do need this, just promise me that you'll do the Whipple Procedure. She said I can't promise that to you.

(This was when she and I had that last minute mini session before she went in to see the doctors .)

And what confirmed it Rossanna, is that we were at UMC (University Medical Center), and a couple of specialists said well, we got good news and bad news. We all said, give us the bad news.

Well, the bad news is that we can't find the growth. And the good news is that typically cancer patients get worse and worse and they progress. You see it in the blood with the samples you take, you see it in the imaging, they won't want to eat, things like that, your mom is showing the opposite." This is of course, after my mom's sessions with you, seeing the doctor in Houston, chi-gong, yoga, meditation, all that stuff.

They were as confused as they could be, and then we found out that they had never performed a Whipple procedure, and they were held back by having my mom go through it because it's a teaching university, and they said, hey, it's a good opportunity to have a teaching moment, and my mom said, the hell with all that!

She said she had nightmares about it, she couldn't talk to my dad about it. I hate that my parents would act that way with you, but she didn't want my dad's family to know. She was scared too, Rossanna, I could so see it, especially not being around for her grandchildren. So it was a very hush-hush thing. And a lot of going to church, things like that, we would pray, we would meditate.

And the thing that you do, I forgot exactly, you know, the tapping. My mom's a little weird about that, but she believed in your sessions, and she told me about them.

She was sick Rossanna, I want you to know she was extremely sick, she was in the hospital, she had so many tests done, I was there all the time, my wife was there, she's a nurse, we talked to the doctors, and they talked about the obstruction in the duct of the pancreas by a mass. They said that she had pancreatic cancer, but yet they could never, after a while, it went away, it went away!

Rossanna, that's the thing, it went away. And that's why they were so, they didn't know what to do! They wanted to know what she did, wanted to know what she was doing, and then my mom just had this, um, distrust of western medicine. She doesn't like it, it's not on her level. I'm so sorry about the mental anguish, the abuse you went through with this.

What I want to say is thank you, because you gave those sessions to her as a gift, you gave my mom peace of mind too, I know that. You know so, I don't know, you're a saint, you really, really are. In my eyes you are. I know that the intention, intentions are what matters, and you had more than intention, you really, really did. I'm glad you reached out to me."

You want to know something? That was all I needed to hear, it was good enough for me. My cousin restored my faith in what really happened 10 years ago. In my heart, I knew she didn't lie, but at the time it occurred, all roads led to that conclusion. I had to sum it all up to make sense of it so I could move on, and I was wrong.

The truth about what happened no longer holds that same sense of urgency for me. What I do know is, in our time together in sessions there was a steady expulsion of negative events and old grudges. And that brought about audible physical relaxation responses every single time. At the same time, she had a prayer going for her, and a shared consciousness of good intentions. She also practiced more than one relaxation method as extra adjunctive therapy. This did not happen from chemotherapy, radiation or radical surgery. In the grander scheme who cares if it was one thing, two, or all of the above? Something happened, and it all worked. I'll let you decide.

Furthermore, at this point in my life, it wasn't about being in a movie after all; that ship had long sailed. It wasn't about having a big successful career, or any of the other things I felt were so important back then. In the end, it's about someone's life.

On a grander scale, I wasn't ready for that type of career back then, it wasn't my time yet. I was a fledgling practitioner, and I had much, much more to learn about the depth of the emotional drivers of serious diseases. Through practical experience, I learned as I went along.

I've had the opportunity to explore and work on every type of illness, disease, and their symptoms, including brain tumors. And also a plethora of cancer presentations, and autoimmune diseases. There is so much I want you to know, and I'll tell you everything I know in my next book, "The Mind-Body Renewal."

And as it turns out, The Angry Pancreas wasn't the great "loose end" for me after all. In reality, it was actually a great "open end" that allowed me to "receive" more information and fine-tune my EFT skills. All so that I could "give" hope to the hard cases, my clients with serious illnesses who continued to seek me out. My acquired approach with EFT was actually the catalyst of something greater. That's what brought me to where I am today. I've got real "street credibility" now, and let me tell you, I earned it. Whew! I am so very grateful for the entire experience, all of it.

The very best thing about it, my aunt is alive and well, living her life on her own terms exactly how she likes it, with her grandchildren all around her. I thank God for that.

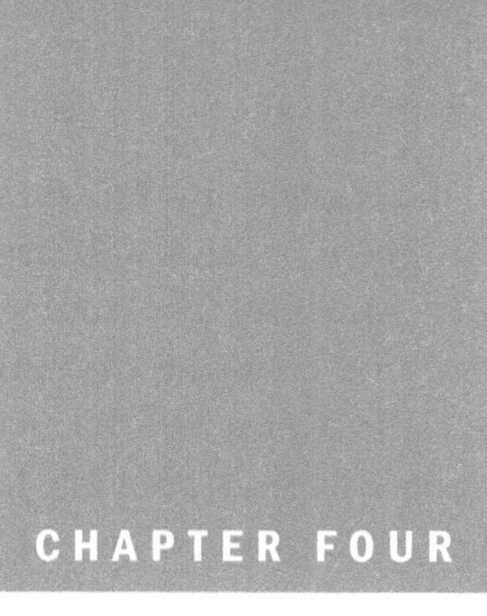

Hello, Stockholm

About a month after all the hoopla died down from my "Angry Pancreas" article, I received a call from Stockholm, Sweden; a woman named Susanne. She read the article. She was diagnosed with pancreatic cancer.

Since that first article, working with people who have pancreatic cancer, or cancer period, has been an unexpected soul journey. What I've learned so far is that not everyone is in alignment with life and the effort to live. The medical profession is aggressive in its approach to treating cancers. But in many ways, they set the stage for failure by creating an attitude of emotional helplessness and hopelessness. In the last fifty years, there has only been a five percent drop in the cancer death rate. And so begins my story about a woman in Sweden named Susanne who decided not to do what she was told and chose instead to live.

We began our work together in August 2008 by phone. In her early sixties, Susanne is an artist, who before her illness loved to paint. She is sensitive, well educated, and a refined woman. Luckily, she is fluent in several languages including English. In brief, she had emotional estrangement issues from both of her parents and had never learned to express anger for fear of more rejection.

Susanne was diagnosed with Stage III pancreatic cancer in June 2004. Stage III means that her cancer had begun to spread and was found in one or more local lymph nodes. They removed part of her pancreas along with the tumor in the standard Whipple procedure. All remaining organs and lymph glands in the area were determined to be clear and healthy. The surgeons called it a successful operation.

As an extra safety measure, she underwent six months of chemotherapy. Told that after enduring the entire traditional medical treatment protocol, she could expect to live at least three years.

Perhaps she was subconsciously obeying her doctor's orders. At precisely the end of her three-year prognosis, she developed a new, "highly aggressive" tumor on what was left of her pancreas. The prognosis was ominous. In fact, her oncologist, when asked about life expectancy, answered: "according to my book you should not be sitting here."

In an attempt to take matters into her own hands, Susanne tried dietary changes from a book by a cancer survivor. Later tests showed no change in her condition. Six months later she began to have severe, unrelenting mid-back pain and was advised to undergo more chemotherapy. This she did for three months until she and her doctor decided to take an eight-week break over the summer so she could travel.

In her mind, she had decided not to resume the treatments but, according to her, didn't know how not to. Under pressure from both her family and her doctor, she had one month before her next CAT scan to determine the extent of her next course of treatments. Intuitively recognizing the need for "deep work" to be done, she sought help energetically through EFT.

But first a word from our sponsor: Energy Psychology.

EFT Cliff Notes

By now, if you're new to "Energy Psychology" and "EFT," you've likely figured out that you say certain phrases while "doing" EFT. So this is a brief overview. Just for you.

Oh, first and foremost it's important to recognize that of all the self-help techniques out there, EFT is the <u>only one</u> that purposely focuses on **negative** thoughts and feelings. I know that seems counter-intuitive, but that's why it works so well!

It calls attention to the way you really feel inside, hitting it head-on minus the sugarcoating. These are the emotional energies you have 'stuck' inside, and the best way to access them for removal is NOT a cover-up positive affirmation. The best way is a straight-on acknowledgment of the negative self-talk running in the background of your mind.

EFT works by tapping on 12 different acupoints on the surface of your body with your fingertips while focusing on **one** specific negative memory or life event.

First, you gauge your emotional 'subjective units of distress' (SUDS) from 0-10 (let's just call it the 'intensity'). Zero is no feeling at all, and ten being the opposite, the high end. The goal is to bring down the emotional intensity to a zero.

This is accomplished by explicitly stating negative feelings and thoughts surrounding that event or memory.

After tapping on the acupoints while stating aloud the negative statements or feelings, you test your results and repeat the process focusing on the same event. You do this until it is completely resolved – zero intensity.

The most methodical approach is to write down specific negative events in your past, in your entire life, one memory at a time. I highly recommend it to everyone if you're serious about real change occurring.

Instead of sitting down and writing a novel about your life as thick as "War and Peace," keep in mind you've already experienced the event. Your mind knows every intricate detail already. Instead, wrap it up (encompass the entire memory) with a couple of words to keep you focused. You'll be surprised by how little you have to say to 'zero-out' the issue.

You simply give each memory a mini-movie title. Starting back as far as you can remember and jot down the intensity of each one (0-10) so you can see your progress. And always bring it down to a zero intensity.

While you're tapping, there's a physical indication that there's been a change or a shift in the way you're feeling about a memory. That's called a physical relaxation response. You might yawn or sigh, or belch. Some people feel tingling sensations throughout their body, feel lighter, calmer, or have a feeling of warmth. And there are other sensations that you can experience.

That's it in a nutshell. In the Appendix, I've gone into detail for those who want to know more. I've also included a history of Energy Psychology/Energy Medicine - quite interesting, really! And references and links, too.

Now, back to Stockholm.

On Your Mark, Get Set, Go!

When we began our sessions Susanne had no appetite, had difficulty eating solid food, was losing weight, and had little or no energy. Because of that, she spent most of her time bedridden not able to leave her house. She was on pain medications that kept the constant pain at a level 4 intensity. Her last blood test results had confirmed her declining state of health, and further impressed on her the desperate nature of her situation.

Starting the race in late August, we had only one month before her next scan. We worked with dizzying intensity twice a week. At the end of our month of sessions, the exams and scans were done. Her oncologist stated that her blood tests were "excellent" and that the cancer had not grown. Susanne herself admitted that she felt a shift back to the way she used to feel before she became ill.

It helped that Susanne was completely open and honest, ready to look at all sides of her life, she was fearless that way. She told me she's spent a lifetime stuffing down emotions, and the only way she could show real anger was to cry. Here are some examples of the phrases used while tapping:

"Even though it's not safe to be myself."

"Even though I always do what I'm told so I can get love and approval."

"Even though I'm very good at being good."

"Even though I'm a terminal cancer patient."

"Even though the research says this cancer is incurable."

"Even though my doctor said I'll never recover."

"Even though I need this cancer for my reasons."

"Even though I don't feel loved unless I'm sick."

"Even though I don't feel special unless I'm sick."

"Even though mother only showed me love and concern when I was sick."

"Even though I don't know how to ask for love unless I manipulate it."

"Even though I'm unworthy of good health, and I don't deserve to get better."

"Even though I need to be rescued, I always have."

Using my "Emotional Trigger-Point Technique," what was the precursor to what I now call "Bitch Tap Method™," I insisted she use words best described as the worst swear words imaginable! I liken it to bursting the emotional balloon of anger.

Once she let loose with what I presumed to be highly colorful language by the tone in which it was delivered (I don't speak Swedish), her back pain went away, eventually completely.

We tapped on her conversations with her doctors, nurses, home health care workers, and anyone else's "dooming" opinions about her illness. As usual, between our set up phrases and tapping rounds, other aspects of her memories tumbled forth. Those quickly led to belching, weakness, rumbling in her stomach, flatulence and even nausea, which always rapidly subsided.

Through my experiences, these seemingly"adverse" reactions are typical with serious health conditions. The body reacts to the energy movement by means of exaggerated physical responses. It still means the same as the more common and benign physical relaxation responses.

We are now approximately five months past her prognostic date with destiny. Our schedule consisted of phone sessions twice a week for three months. Then we tapered off to once a week with email interactions and homework during the week - technically still twice a week.

So far, Susanne is still firm in her decision not to resume her scheduled chemo treatments. She's gone from bedridden and barely able to walk from her bed to her kitchen, to taking a weekend trip with a girlfriend for a holiday of painting.

Her appetite graduated from only certain soft foods to a variety of solids, and now even cooks for herself. Although she no longer feels constant pain, her fear of it coming back has caused her to continue taking her pain medications. But she has tapered her dose and reports that she's still without pain. So intensive was our work together that she experienced two months of what she, at the time, described as exhaustion. Now, later, she describes it as a deep, much-needed rest. She recognizes it intuitively as part of her healing process and feels very different now because of it. She says her changes are now noticeably evident to her friends and family, who say she has a lighter spirit about her.

Susanne says "I have the feeling that I somehow am in charge of my body and my health and that has been truly empowering." And after spending so many years silently angry and resentful at both of her parents, she says that if she were to have a second chance, she would choose them both again. She also expressed gratitude for the extraordinary life they afforded her. She said that if she did have that second chance, she would instead change HER attitude toward them. Based on our work together I found these shifts to clarity and forgiveness to be particularly rewarding.

Admittedly, we've both agreed we are far from through with our work together. This article is intended to let you know how far we've come with EFT and the emotions behind this type of cancer. Suffice it to say that so far, as she was told by her oncologist, who is known not to dispense false hope, her current lab reports are entirely normal! When the Oncologist went over her newest test results, she exclaimed to Susanne, and I quote: "You don't understand, this is fantastic"! Also stating that her once very aggressive tumor is now "inactive" as if the ignition switch had been turned off! In fact, since they can no longer find the tumor, the doctors have decided it must be "hiding" behind something. Since starting on writing this article, she has undergone yet another round of tests with the same excellent conclusions.

While she is not out of the woods yet, there are fewer trees, and they are smaller, apparently receding into the distance. A Stage III pancreatic cancer considered "operable" still has only a 20% survival rate at five years, and much, much less if there is a recurrence. Even though she was under appropriate, conventional medical care, the predicted outcome was not good.

Based on our results, there's a high probability that the changes in the outcome so far have something to do with the clearing of life-threatening negative emotional energies, i.e., EFT.

Surviving a recurrence of Stage III is uncommon, much less its apparent "remission" and return toward health. If the future continues as brightly as the recent past progress, then Susanne will set a new standard as a proactive participant in her own healing. Adding Emotional healing to every aspect covers all bases.

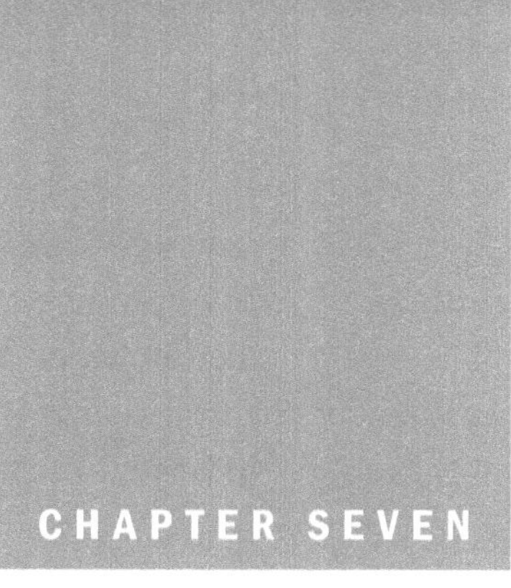

The Trade-Off

Susanne's story of emotional recovery and positive physical response was affirming and exciting.

I was gearing up to write the sequel of her life after cancer, but it wasn't meant to be. It has literally taken me nine years to finally put into words and finish the second half of this story. It's still incredible to me. Even several thousand client experiences later, I can honestly say, I still feel the same way about the outcome.

For several months, Susanne was physically asymptomatic. She was back to painting, traveling, cooking, eating well, and doing exactly what she loved to do.

Our sessions continued to decrease from once a month, to her just checking in with me for a quick chat about current events and new happenings in her life. Her daughter, Olivia, had recently given birth, a little girl, her new granddaughter. She felt joyful and anticipated the future. She also dutifully continued her daily EFT self-work with the special homework assignments at her request that I provided for her. We continued to mark her progress.

Her last hurdle overcome was the morphine, given to terminally ill patients for pain, but highly addictive. The general medical mindset is who care's if it's addictive, at least they won't feel pain, and they're dying anyway which makes sense. Now that she proved them wrong, it was a reality she had to deal with next.

With her oncologist's guidance, she reduced her daily dosage and was actively working to wean herself off of it all together.

Sometime later, ever the inquisitive seeker of new knowledge, Susanne had a reading with a renowned Scandinavian psychic and health intuitive. We consulted in a later phone call about the meaning. The psychic told her: "I see you covered in water, surrounded by water." Susanne wondered if that meant she would drown? I saw it as a possible health-related metaphor. Neither one of us knew at the time, but we would both be right.

And then one evening I received a call from Susanne, who sounded like she had been crying. The tone of her voice seemed very weak, a breathless, punched in the solar plexus pain wracked voice, I knew something was terribly wrong.

On the drive back to Stockholm after a family holiday, Susanne's daughter, Olivia, developed a dry cough that severely worsened. After thorough medical examinations and diagnostic studies, Olivia was told she had an "inoperable" and "incurable" lung tumor. The prognostic guess was very grim, a matter of months at best.

That was the last conversation I would ever have with Susanne. She spoke of how unfair it was that Olivia, a new mother, would never experience the profound joys of motherhood as she had. She remarked that she had already lived a long, full and wonderful life, how beautiful it has been, and how much love she's known through it all. Now her beautiful young daughter had a death sentence. "It isn't fair; it's not supposed to happen this way, why her? Why can't it be me? It isn't fair."

When I heard her say that, I knew how this would end.

And so it was, I learned very soon afterward, Susanne's health gave way. Her entire body swelled with fluids, and she quietly drifted off into a coma. She never revived. I remembered the drowning water, the health-related metaphor from her psychic reading earlier.

Before she passed away our mutual friend in Sweden went to pay his respects to her family, and say goodbye to her. He told me about his visit and said; "It's the strangest thing, but she has the most peaceful, the most beautiful smile on her face."

From this experience, and with the "untimely" death of my brother in the early eighties as a contrast, my personal beliefs about death and dying had shifted into something less fearful and ominous, into just being another extension of life. Death is not a punishment for those who pass, or for the ones they leave behind, and it's not the worst thing that could happen to you. No matter the circumstance, it's always meant to be exactly that way, at exactly the right time, whether anyone is ready for it or not.

I can now say that from my years of work with the seriously ill, I learned a valuable lesson. I know now that the worst thing that could happen to you is to die without peace in your heart. The worst thing is a conscience filled with old grudges and regrets because you weren't awake enough to rectify things while you still had the opportunity.

It seems that in the order of importance in the treatment of serious illnesses, emotional healing has largely been overlooked. In fact, it's underplayed.

Almost fifty percent of the people I've accepted as clients had stage 4 cancers. They contact me after spending a great deal of precious time and money going through other treatments. By the time they get to me, their physical decline had gone beyond the point of recovery. Those are the cases that turn out to be more of an EFT "hospice" practice. Their healing comes in the form of self-acceptance, resolution, forgiveness, and deep personal peace. I even had a last minute speed-dial deathbed session with one client. I'll talk more about Hospice EFT in an upcoming book.

It's my opinion that emotional recovery should be first in line at the first diagnosis. It's something you can do for yourself while you're waiting to go through other treatments. That step in the right direction makes you immediately proactive. You're doing something about it, not waiting for someone to do it for you. As for prevention, there's no stronger medicine than EFT.

Susanne had combed through every negative aspect of her life and found clarity and forgiveness while we were together. I knew that. Contrary to my religious upbringing and past beliefs, even though her death was imminent, I felt no sadness about it whatsoever. I felt calm, even tranquil. And I knew why she was smiling.

It was at dusk when I received the call that she was gone. I walked outside that evening to see an artist's sky, the most dramatic purple and orange sunset I've ever seen. Sitting alone on the porch steps, I looked up to bid her farewell, honoring her existence and paid homage to the most beautiful legacy she left behind. She was done with this place, and she was satisfied.

With the deepest gratitude, I'd like to acknowledge her family and friends for keeping me informed during that time. I am forever grateful for their kindness and of the generosity of their time communicating with me.

I was moved to write a tribute to her in time for the funeral service. It was read to the congregation by a renown Lutheran Scandinavian priest officiating the funeral.

Tribute to Susanne

By Dr. Rossanna Massey

It is with great admiration and respect that I pay tribute today to my friend Susanne.

Although it's impossible to summarize such an extraordinary life, I feel honored to give you my impression of her.

Although Susanne was a very unpretentious and unassuming woman, she came from privilege. She was a world traveler who had a natural propensity for learning many languages with great ease and agility. Susanne was what we call in America a Maverick. A non-conformist who dared to be different while others played it safe. She lived a very rich and colorful life laced with a soulful passion in all of her endeavors. She was naturally drawn to the quest for spiritual enlightenment and inner peace. It is my belief she achieved that in her lifetime. As I was told by her family and friends in her final days, it was evident by her apparent serenity.

Beyond her obviously, beautiful physicality was the soul of an artist and a woman who loved very passionately, and very deeply. She was very sensitive and intuitive to the feelings and needs of others, often to her detriment. With all her heart, Susanne loved her family and friends, and the father of her children, Daniel, with graceful humanity and a full-hearted kinship of loyalty.

Yet, nothing can fully describe or compare to the way she felt about her two children, Olivia, and Peter. If I can be of comfort to you at this very moment, I would say that your presence and the privilege of being your mother made her life complete. And that she was extremely proud of you and the way you were both able to express your lives as freely as she expressed hers. It was the highlight of her life to have both Julia and Paula grace her with the fullness of love that only grandchildren can give. She could only best describe them as beautiful.

I will forever miss her lovely lyrical voice, her beautiful and free spirit, her candid narrations of life in Sweden. Our friendship was one based on faith in the human spirit. We never met in person, yet I am so connected to her even now, that I can hardly bring myself to feel her loss just yet. I prefer to keep her memory as if encased as a beautifully wrapped present waiting to be open. Her friendship was a gift to me that I shall always treasure very dearly. I will never forget the brilliance of her presence or the impression that she made in my life for as long as I live.

God keep you by his side dearest Susanne. Go in peace, my darling friend.

Darling friend, you say? The only thing I can tell you is that when I work with someone, especially for this long, I've seen their entire life story unfold in my mind's eye as we tap. I can see, feel, hear the real them before, during and after the wounds. It's always such an honor to be trusted to that extent. Viewing their life-reel, I can see who they are, that person, and to know them truly is to love them. You just can't help but love an innocent little child. It feels so primary and simple, yet, I find it hard to explain. I don't see it as a problem for me because it means I'm present energetically, right in the moment. And that makes for a highly productive and successful session.

I eventually taught myself how to shake off client energy with EFT, so it never lingers with me. I'm in love with the essence of all my clients. What they do with that essence, right or wrong, I can also let go of when our work is complete. Even so, I can see the person they always were. The beautiful, innocent little children they were inside, all grown up now, navigating through life as best they can. It's very beautiful, and an honor I will forever respect and never take for granted.

Until now, aside from my husband, George, I never shared her story. I tucked her file away thinking perhaps one day, but not then, I'd have the courage to open it back up and go through it all again to finish it. At the time it happened, it felt too big to try and explain it to anyone, so I never did. So much time has passed between us since then, I no longer feel that way. See a pattern? Too big=overwhelm, can't put into words. Lol! It's been the focus of my self-work!

I've always loved a happy ending, and I'm delighted to say this story ends with one. Nine years later, Susanne's daughter, Olivia, is alive, thriving, traveling, and raising her daughter. It's everything Susanne had ever hoped and prayed for.

Like her mother, Olivia listened to her inner wisdom and said no to most of the invasive medical procedures offered as her only options. Instead, she only agreed to cutting edge, noninvasive cancer treatments, including EFT sessions with me to address the emotional layer of healing. She still only follows what resonates with her mind and her body for self-care, and she lives happily ever after.

Rude Awakening

My path to self-improvement meant I had to learn how to be open and receptive to new information. That meant me not feeling threatened and throwing rocks at the things I didn't yet know about. Even if they did look crazy and I doubted it, at least I would try it. Boy, I was in for a rude awakening! I wasn't an easy nut to crack, but fortunately for me, I had a very good teacher, literally. (Shut up Wendi!) Lol!

It all starts with a certain Dr. George A. Massey, the most precious and most beloved person in my life. In the early 70's he was a senior instructor for Jose Silva in "Silva Mind Control." His extensive background in hypnotherapy and alternative healing methods was a huge influence. Through George's experience and knowledge, I learned new healing concepts both esoteric and traditional therapies. Those extra jewels of wisdom gave me the added advantage of keeping me fresh and on point clinically. I have so much gratitude and respect for him and his wisdom. He and I met and fell madly in love during my last quarter of Chiropractic college in California. He asked me to marry him on our third date and I said yes.

After graduation, I started off as an associate doctor in a large Hispanic clinic in the Mission District of San Francisco. As if it fell into our laps, (meant to be) we found an established private practice for sale in Southwest Michigan. The big surprise was that was also only

30 minutes away from where I grew up! So there I was, after almost 20 years of self-exile from my hometown. I moved back to the Midwest and took George with me.

We settled in Bridgman, Michigan. It's a beautiful, cozy, lakeside town located in the southwest part of the state. Our office was surrounded by the ever-changing lush foliage of the woodlands. It had large picture windows that gave us beautiful, seasonal panoramic views. We called ourselves "The Bridgman Chiropractors."

We loved our patients, and we knew they loved us back. Not only did they entrust us with their lives and their health, but they also had faith in us. Together we practiced the latest, cutting-edge adjunctive therapies to complement mind/body health. We offered clinical hypnotherapy, nutritional protocols, and detoxifications to improve vitality. Our patients eagerly came along for the benefit.

It was our patients who taught me how to connect the emotional dots with health problems. Since then I've gotten so good at it (I teach you emotional trends in our next book) that I can go there in seconds. I zero in on the emotional drivers of a health problem as soon as I hear it. It even happens if a person tells me about their health issues in passing. This is my life's work - it's the way I'm wired to think, I'm expert at it.

Through the years I got to know our patient's personal histories. I knew their joys, sorrows, divorces, disappointments and their anger. I could feel, see, hear the way they viewed themselves, and see how it affected their health issues. The less self-love, and self-compassion they had, the more relentless at punishing themselves. That meant ignoring and pushing themselves past physical pain. And when your body is trying to tell you something is wrong through the language of pain, you should care enough to stop and listen.

These were the patients who were strictly symptom oriented. They would only come in for treatment after they couldn't stand it anymore. What was worse, they had the nerve to be impatient for the time it took to heal properly. I grew to understand the enormity of emotional trends. They directly influence acute and chronic pain syndromes. In fact, that goes for any health issue, cancer included. The global name of the trigger is otherwise known as "stress." It was one thing for me to recognize it because I learned there was a predictable pattern. It was before I knew EFT even existed, so I just didn't know what to do about it yet.

George subscribed to a popular nutritional website and glanced through it daily. On there he saw a link for "Emotional Freedom Techniques, (EFT). The founder, Gary Craig, offered a free download of his how-to manual and an introductory video. What really impressed him was that Gary was giving this information away for free! In Gary's own words, he wanted the world to know about EFT. His altruistic approach of "gifting" was absolutely unheard of at the time. What, no profit? A donation if we'd like? What the heck?

As George would tell it, he downloaded the manual, skimmed through it once, and thought it looked silly. He set it down without looking at it for two years.

Unbeknown to me, he picked it up again and pulled it out of his bag of clinical tricks! He used it on one of his patients, a single mom with a puzzling problem. She was a housekeeper, working long hours doing physical labor, came in for mid back and neck pain. On her last visit, she was so happy to be feeling a million times better.

During treatment, George found her muscles exceptionally tight and tender in her upper-mid back and informed her that this region of the spine affects the stomach and intestines. He told her the treatment should help with her digestion.

As she was getting up from the treatment table she said; "Oh good, maybe that will help with my throwing up every day. I've been throwing up every morning for the last 17 years starting after the birth of my son, I throw up every morning. Sometimes it's just dry heaves, but most of the time something comes up. After I throw up I'm fine. I get up and get everyone ready for school, make breakfast, but my family knows it's just the thing I do. I've seen a bunch of doctors about it over the years, nothing worked."

George claims to have spent 5-10 minutes with her in his treatment room maybe doing 3 rounds of tapping. He walked her out to the quiet common area with only a staff member, and I, at the front desk.

To make sure she remembered how to do it, he demonstrated the tapping sequence with her again. He had her say weird things in front of us like "I accept myself even though I have this problem." There they were, tapping away, knocking on their heads, face, chest, and fingers. I swore I'd never seen anything look so ridiculous, are you kidding me? Was he really just making this up as he went along? I stood there thinking to myself "you look nutty doing this, George. Okay, you should stop now, where in the heck did you find this goofy stuff at anyway?" It looked crazy to me, whaddya mean meridians? Huh?

As soon as she left, I asked what the heck just happened? George said, "I was trying something new I picked up on the internet to see if it worked." I love that about him!

We ran into her at the grocery store later in the week. The minute she saw us she said; "Hey guess what doc, I haven't thrown up since we did that!" George and I were both plucked! You're kidding. Really?

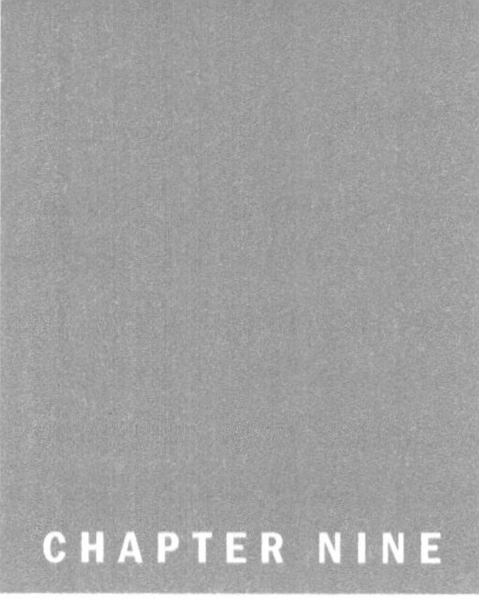

I "Got It"

Two weeks later she came to the clinic for a follow-up. She exclaimed that it has been a good three weeks since she last threw up in the morning!

There was a core issue released by the new tapping technique. By saying; "This problem," she had actually "tapped" into a major negative time in her life. And this issue was her subconscious priority.

It was the time when she was pregnant and abandoned by her baby's daddy. It was "stuck" inside her stomach! The emotional remnant of that fearful realization never went away. She literally took it in the gut. She was truly alone in this situation, completely on her own. It made her puke, and she didn't stop her morning ritual of "rise and Ralph" for the next 17 years.

For years she had sought both medical and psychological help. But none of them could find anything wrong. There was still no diagnostic cause.

This was a miraculous recovery!

This patient would be my George's EFT one-minute wonder! Subsequent follow-ups with her further verified EFT had indeed worked its wonders. What is this stuff anyway?

Okay, now that caught my attention. So I tried something crazy like EFT. I read the EFT manual myself. And I read it again, and again.

I started out with a healthy dose of intellectual resistance. I figured this stuff had to be a bunch of bologna. But the minute I tried it and collapsed my very first issue, EFT clicked with me right away.

I still love to muse about working on my very first EFT tapping issue. It was a mixture of disbelief and wonderment. My first thoughts were; wait a minute, where did that just go? (I'm very visual) Hey, what just happened? Holy cow! You gotta be kidding me! No way! Huh, how do you like that? It's the memories of me trying it in the early years that always keeps me connected and excited for the newbies to EFT. I totally get it. Sigh, I know, right?

I have no better explanation for it except that I just "got" how it worked immediately afterward. I was completely driven to keep doing it on myself. I had absolutely no problem with follow through. Per the free EFT manual, I created my own Personal Peace Procedure list. I added every traumatic event and negative memory I could think of. But I "omitted" all the past events "I already worked on" with my therapist back in California (more about that later). Those I thought were done, resolved, and non-issues now. Yeah, right!

I was compelled to give it the benefit of the doubt; it was too good to be true. What if it really did work? But each painful scene of every bad event ever I went through, broke apart in my mind's eye and went away. I couldn't piece the fragments of the memory back together again. It was all very odd, very different, and all gone with not even the slightest emotional charge left over. As if the weights lifted, the heavy luggage, set down. It's that strange feeling when you've been lifting heavy weights and your arms feel light and a little shaky? It was that kinesthetic feeling. I felt lighter. And I felt better. Cleaning out your past brings you back in touch with the innocent little kid you started out being. Now you're a hell of a lot wiser, yet no worse for the wear. Get it?

One negative memory at a time, I knocked off my list. Very soon it was one side of the page off my list after the other, onto the next page. The older the memories were, the faster they fell away. The bigger and more common theme of the memory, the more similar ones fell away along with it. It was like playing pinball and winning every shot. Like bowling and knocking down all the pins at once, hitting a strike every time!

I tried EFT on absolutely everything just to see how far I could take it. I even used it on myself for acute injuries like kitchen accidents and everyday stuff. Finally, I had the idea to focus on and test all the things

I worked on with my therapist in Chiropractic college. It was the stuff I omitted from my initial list. I mean why not? Just for the hell of it.

When I guesstimated each intensity level, it always felt very low, a 1 or a 2 at most if at all. But for testing sake, I tapped on every single one of them anyway. Boom! Time and again, there they were, just like it happened yesterday! The tears came so quickly, the tightening in my throat, the tightening in my chest. There they were, the residual cellular emotional response waiting for an exit. That was enough evidence for me to fully comprehend that we're not done with this stuff in talk therapy. Not until the energy it created has exited the body. This means, although it may seem so intellectually, it's not enough to just talk about your problem. There must also be an accompaniment of negative energy released. It's as if it comes from inside the tissues at a cellular level and exits through an acupoint. That's when you're completely done with it physically...and emotionally.

My own results with EFT were so clean, it literally took me about three months to fully wrap my head around it. It took me that long to realize how powerful EFT was. And at least that long to register how my entire outlook on life began to shift for the better. And I'm delighted to say, I'm still a work in progress. No special ivory tower seating going on up in here! Lol!

I had to know more about EFT. The more I did, the more I realized my life was about to go off into a different trajectory. I was about to shift into a profession I know with every fiber of my being, I was born to do. I had paid tens of thousands of dollars for my professional education, but it no longer mattered. The truth known, career-wise, I knew I was on the right track as a holistic doctor, but it didn't feel like it fit just right. And that form of healing didn't superimpose over my new, current vision. Even our beloved office manager, Carol (aka Lil Carol) could pick up on it intuitively. She would make comments to me about my heart not being into it. Sigh. I heard you girl, you were right!

During that time, I read anything I could get my hands on that Gary Craig wrote. I read every article by other practitioners, and I watched every single video he had more than once. I made it a point to attend every workshop possible.

My patients trusted me, and I was fortunate that they allowed me to practice EFT on them during their visits. We tapped for their serious diseases, chronic pain syndromes, and even acute conditions. I even worked with my husband's patients, especially the ones who seemed to be mystery cases. All with unbelievable success and obvious results, hundreds of them. It was mind-blowing.

I set my sights on entering the EFT Master's certification program. As a physician with years of clinical experience under my wing, I knew my area of specialty. I would specialize in the emotional drivers of Serious Diseases and Pain Syndromes. The first steps were to earn my Beginner and Advanced EFT certificate of completion. I achieved those in succession and kept my focus on my ultimate goal.

One of many requirements to become an EFT Master was that I had to relinquish any other profession. That meant I had to work strictly as an EFT practitioner for three years before entering the program. It was an easy career decision for me to make, no doubt about it. After 17 years of clinical practice, I retired from Chiropractic, but I still retain my license.

A prerequisite from the very beginning for any level of EFT practitioner was that we work on our own issues.

That is the responsible thing to do if we're putting ourselves out there to help other people. It's optimal for the client's recovery that their sessions be all about them. A top-notch practitioner is one who's own filters are clear. Clarity keeps you present when you're in a session with a client. You're not offering clarity if you're jaded by similar unresolved past experiences. Those thoughts will influence the direction of the session. It's not therapeutic, and it's confusing to the client.

My professional decision to retire left George working the Chiropractic end of things. With his help, I made an office for myself as an "Advanced Practitioner" at the clinic seeing EFT clients.

I'm so grateful for the time we had in Michigan because it was the best practical experience I could ever have. I had a built-in, steady sample of every type of disease and health condition present to me in person. And it also provided frequent follow-ups in person. Being naturally fearless, I took it all on. It was my incubation period of sorts.

I tried EFT on everything. In my sales pitch, I would tell our patients that they had nothing to lose but a little pain. We gave them an offer they couldn't refuse! Such a deal! For the sake of science and exploration, almost every single patient graciously accepted.

CHAPTER TEN

Metaphors, Anyone?

It's been a great opportunity to practice EFT on patients with a variety of health conditions. I'm fascinated by the use of metaphors as a subliminal, coded language that speaks to the body, and how the body interprets them as if it already knows. Here is an interesting example of one.

Andrea was a quiet, soft-spoken woman with left-sided facial numbness for twelve years. She was George's regular patient. Although a very skilled clinician, nothing he did seemed to address it for very long.

At my first exposure to EFT, I realized the significance of emotional healing and how it affects the body. As a bonus to my patients, I incorporated it into my practice on a regular basis. I was particularly interested in experimenting with metaphors. My husband suggested to Andrea that she try something new. Since she had nothing to lose but a little time and numbness, she agreed to a session with me.

Andrea determined that her facial numbness intensity was a 6. Here's how it unfolded. "Even though the left side of my face is numb, and it's been numb for so long, I doubt it will go away, I deeply and profoundly accept who I am." After the first round, I could tell she was more relaxed, and the numbness decreased to a 4. Before we began the second round she said; "My husband has a drinking problem, and I feel trapped because he won't stop." I asked her how long he's been that way, she said ever since they lost their business twelve years ago. I asked how she dealt with it daily and was intrigued by her response. "I turn my face to it because there's nothing I can do to change it, and I don't want to break up my family." My intuition kicked in with our next tapping round, and the setup phrase went as follows. "Even though I can't face the past, present, or future, I deeply and profoundly accept myself." The numb face for twelve years had disappeared completely after only two rounds of EFT!

Andrea was shocked and quite happy with her results. But now she could see her situation more clearly and knew where it could lead. She declined a follow-up session because she was afraid it would make her divorce her husband. I accepted that as her deep truth and understood it. Recognizing her fear of change, I knew it wasn't my place to rescue her either. It was only about the numbness.

I often times ponder karmic realities. Why do some of us take an active role in growth opportunities and some pass it by? Do we settle into bad situations for life lessons or is it only us being locked into fear? Awake, or asleep?

In all honesty, after this session, Andrea went as far as avoiding eye contact with me. She "revealed" herself in her session, actually said it out loud, and now, for her own reasons, it was back to reality. Her true feelings held back, it was better not to feel anything at all about what she was "facing" in her life. She eventually stopped coming in for Chiropractic treatments.

Knowing how deeply EFT can resonate, in this case it was a catalyst for new realizations for Andrea. I trust that our session did something to awaken, and on some level confirm her true feelings. At the very least, Andrea could now connect the dots to her facial symptoms. Did the problem of the numb face come back after that? I'll never know, but I hope she found the strength to resolve her marital problem.

CHAPTER ELEVEN

From The Ashes

I kept plugging away, writing and publishing articles based on clinical experiences. I helped more and more people by refining my approaches to health and physical symptoms.

George and I grew tired of the cold weather, gray skies, snow shoveling, and the adverse winter conditions. After a lovely vacation in the land of enchantment, New Mexico, we decided to leave Michigan. In love with the warmer, sunnier climate we came home and put our house and our practice up for sale and waited.

Soon afterward the state of Michigan began its economic descent into dire straits. Worse yet, real estate sales began to bottom out as the economy took the giant nose-dive. That caused big and small established businesses in Bridgman to close their doors. George did his best dealing with decreased patient numbers at the clinic. I saw EFT clients on the internet at home to help us keep afloat. It was during that time I had sessions with "Karen" from the Angry Pancreas story.

After three years and six different real estate agents, there were a few lookers but no bites. We had a close call with our clinic that didn't turn out, but nothing on our house. Our practice slowly shrank before our eyes. Before we knew it, we were unable to keep up with the clinic expenses and make our house payments at the same time. At the advice of our trusted accountant, who delivered the devastating news, we had to let go of both. George and I sold off our clinic records and equipment, and let our house go into foreclosure.

One evening, searching on Craig's list for rental properties, I discovered a new listing. It was a beautiful adobe hacienda in Anthony, New Mexico, very close to El Paso. It boasted panoramic views of three different mountain ranges from the great room. It had a grand hallway, and a big Spanish-tiled water fountain in the middle of the courtyard. An added bonus was a casita (small guest house) situated across the expansive veranda.

The owner was a tenured college professor of physics who was raised in Mexico. So it was traditionally made from handmade adobe mud bricks made on site. That meant it was naturally able to withstand the desert climate. The hacienda was strategically placed at the top of the mesa for optimal sun exposure year round. It was calculated into position to keep it cool in the summer and warm in the winter.

The hacienda was on ten acres. Behind it was over two hundred thousand acres of government property. It was so isolated that not everyone was willing to live up there. Lucky for us, the rent reflected that as well. George was suspicious, it all sounded too good to be true. I thought the pictures of the place were convincing.

Special thanks to my wonderful, one and only little sister, Diana, for this part of the story! Already living nearby in ElPaso, she offered to see the place for us to make sure it wasn't a scam. She met with a property manager who asked her to follow his car up the mesa. I stayed on the phone with her in case the guy was a crook with bad intentions. At the foot of the mesa, she set out to drive up the steep, sandy slope, saying; "Oh my God" its kind of scary." As she drove up the mesa's winding dirt road, she was pensive. I'll never forget her words the minute she parked her car and walked up to the courtyard. "Oh my God!" Then she walked into the hacienda and a got a load of the views, "OH MY GOD!" That did it! We rented it sight unseen. What belongings we couldn't sell before we left Michigan, George and I gave away.

Our moving truck packed, our two dogs and four cats in tow waiting for us in the car, we took one last walk through our house. It was the place of so many wonderful memories, the first home I ever owned; we both worked so hard on it, inside and out. We stood in the middle of our living room and said our goodbyes, each of us recalling a special happy memory aloud. We used EFT and tapped for not being able to let go of our home. Guess what? It turns out, we could let go after all.

Walking away with our backs to the house, and our faces to the future, we climbed into our vehicles, and headed southwest. Homeward bound to the Land of Enchantment, New Mexico, the hacienda, and our new beginning. From the ashes arise the Phoenix.

Fort Bummer

Our little welcome wagon to Anthony, New Mexico, was a splendid welcome home. It consisted of my loving, benevolent Tio (uncle) Jaime, and his wife, my Tia (aunt) Alice. With their three grown children and their spouses, they helped us unload, unpack, and settle in. And they brought food, lots of food because that's exactly how my Mexican family rolls! I love them all so much for their selflessness, and their kindness for the time they spent with us. Actually, more than one of my mother's siblings would later step up to lend a hand. I have a deep love, respect and appreciation for all the ways my tios and tias represented. Los amo mucho a todos.

For that matter, our earlier years at the hacienda are worthy of their own book, which I still plan on writing one day. It was our place of healing, our private retreat. Along with our friends and family, we shared many a moonlight night partying on the big veranda. We played music, and sang songs, and howled at the moon with the coyotes in the candlelight. It was a wonderful, and magical gathering place, making it natural to host dinner parties. It was there that we met our two best friends. Accomplished chefs, they had a beautiful little "farmette" right below the mesa from us. And can they cook, and bake! Trust me, when their dinner bell rings, we drop everything and come running! There were times together we would imagine having a zip line to and from the top of the mesa to their house! Did I mention we had fun living there? OMG!

Career-wise, my internet business kept us going in Anthony. I was seeing private and local clients while working my way closer to my goal of becoming an EFT Master. Three months before completing all my prerequisites, Gary Craig closed the Master's program. My Intermediate Academic Certification Level II was the closest I could ever get to it. I'm still very proud I made it that far because I earned it. I had learned from the master himself.

Mom's closest sister, my Tia Elma, and her husband, Tio Gus, have a very well-connected family business in El Paso. My wonderful cousins (their children) provided us with the unique opportunity to present EFT at the large Army base in El Paso, Fort Bliss. At the time their PTSD problems on base were no secret and actually were intensifying. Our goal was to open the discussion for trying EFT as a different approach.

Ugh, doggone it, we bombed miserably. With a background in radio, and years of teaching, George's public speaking skills were on point (so proud). But I was the one with no experience, I can own this one for sure.

They presented me with two volunteers whom I knew nothing about. They pre-agreed to tap (which they knew nothing about) in front of an audience. The pressure that we both felt for different reasons was insurmountable. I hadn't thought out the logistics of our presentation to be at my advantage.

Bringing up someone I'd never met before reduced my performance to a ridiculous circus act. It was horrifying to be in the position of hurry-up and produce real-time drama and pronto! They were looking for that wow factor they couldn't ignore! Gulp.

When I thought about this later, could I blame my subjects for what happened? What soldier wants commanding officers and strangers see them break down and cry like a baby? What if this stuff made them feel too vulnerable? In full uniform, they stood stoic, each with their own challenging, dueling stares. I felt as if they were daring me to crack their nut. In fact, I knew they were.

And there you have it, surrounded by clinic directors, clinicians, and the top brass of Fort Bliss. I floundered, I bombed, I blew it. The wall of veteran resistance was as thick and resistant as iron. An iron wall ten feet thick, wrapped in barbed wire. Sigh.

I could just kick myself for feeling so honored to be there, and too beholding for the huge favor! I didn't want to "rock the boat" and appear too pushy. I was too afraid to take command (pun intended) of the situation and call the shots on how I wanted the presentation. I should have told them what I required beforehand to showcase EFT in the best possible way. Duh! Lol!

Worse yet, it took that face to face moment with the veterans for me to realize my biggest disadvantage. I failed to discuss the possibility of our results taking more time to happen due to medications. I should have insisted upon brief initial consultations. It would also help me determine who I could work with given their issues within an hour presentation.

It's exactly what I do with a private client before I begin their sessions. I missed my opportunity to ask each veteran in private ahead of time if they were on medications, if so, how much?

In front of everyone, it was too late to do that. As a doctor doing so in public without their permission ahead of time would be a violation of their privacy. Psychotropic drugs act as an energy toxin that dulls and stall the results of tapping. It doesn't stop results, it just takes more effort and time for it to happen. It was actually THE most important question I failed to ask. This was my one shot, and I had precious little time to show them some big results. There I was, stuck in front of an audience, and I had just embarrassed myself publicly. Ugh! But I kept my cool. Things happen for a reason. I wasn't ready yet.

Believe it or not, I still received private referrals after this presentation. I grew to understand the more complexed details of the layers of PTSD. I could see why some have it worse than others, and some not at all. Like Postpartum depression, it's an anxiety overload. The amount of anxiety you had before the "new" negative events adds to the load and turns into overload.

CHAPTER THIRTEEN

Baby Blues

I'm very fortunate that I have family members who trust and support my work. It's not always the case, as some of you practitioners out there may know. One of mom's brothers, and his wife, actually attended one of my EFT workshops! After learning the power and potential of EFT, they sought my help for their daughter.

I have long wondered why there was such a mixed bag of experiences for women post postpartum. How is it that some women get depressed and others do not? Is it just an unbalanced internal chemical mix that happens randomly? Or are there contributing emotional factors to ignite it? What gives a woman the propensity to not be able to handle a normal hormonal shift after delivery?

I had my chance to finally work with a willing participant, a close cousin of mine. She had delivered her second son, one week before our first session. She had severe postpartum depression following the birth of her first son. She said it was so severe that she was only able to breastfeed her son and then immediately hand him over to her husband. She couldn't handle much more than that. She was prescribed the anti-depression medication, Zoloft one month after she gave birth. According to her, it did nothing to reduce the symptoms.

Her "overwhelm" began shortly after she gave birth until July of the following year for a total of 13 months!

At the birth of her new son, knowing what happened with her first child, the family waited for the other shoe to drop. It did with a vengeance.

I paid a visit to my cousin for our first session. She had been crying all morning. After I gave her instruction on how and where to tap, I asked her how she felt in the moment as a place of reference. The only thing she could say was "I can't do this" (referring to being a mother to two small children at once). So, we started with: "Maybe I can accept myself even though I can't do this." After the first round of tapping, her anxiety levels dropped dramatically. She knew right away this was good for her, and we were onto something! She became one of my most motivated subjects and didn't shy away from any issue in her past. She wanted nothing more than to get beyond these moods and get on with being the best mom she could be.

For the duration of our sessions, we worked very well together. I guessed the duration of treatments and decided on an hour session daily for two weeks. During that time we uncovered layers of traumatic childhood events. It all began with being bullied in grade school numerous times. Those issues lead us to even more bullying events in high school by the "mean girls" on campus. She also had a strong sibling rivalry dynamic with an older sibling. Since she's the baby of the family, she got picked on by him, which in essence turned into serial bullying at home.

Through it all my cousin never told anyone what she was going through in school or at home. It was an understandable non-reaction for her own self-preservation--for fear of repercussion.

Other fear-inducing memories included a frightening auto accident and a Peeping Tom episode. Here's a side note about the Peeping Tom: I noticed that she always kept her drapes and blinds closed in her house. At the time I thought it was very peculiar, but I had a hunch about it--turns out I was right. She was still afraid of someone looking in her windows. By the way...she now keeps the windows uncovered during the day and lets the sunshine in!

Her feelings of powerlessness, helplessness and inadequacy stemmed from unexpressed, stuffed-down emotions. Energetically, holding all that down causes a combustible vibrational imbalance called "anxiety." The anger and sadness she felt from those experiences turned into "depression."

Her physical relaxation responses and their locations during our tapping were not surprising. In fact, they fit with her emotional issues as they always do. The symptoms would manifest in her throat, it would get tight, (afraid to speak). Once we removed the fear from her throat and used "Bitch Tap," it would relax. Some issues gave her chest wall tension until the issue resolved. Other times she would belch which was our clear indication she was over yet another issue. FYI, all areas of reaction corresponded to the underlying Chakras (energy centers) involved. In my next book, "Mind Body Renewal" I go over this concept in great detail as it relates to your health. As "emotional catchers mitts" Chakras catch and hang onto negative and traumatic events. They also catch and hang onto positive events. The location where each issue is stored dictates the area of a physical reaction.

To my delight, my cousin was willing to find time for daily intensive sessions for as long as it took. And that's what it takes for fast, and positive change to occur. We managed to get through her Storyboard procedure in twelve days! The last two days we were literally fishing for straws to find things to work on, so we focused on a different family issue. Since it helped her so much, she knew it could help her little son too.

My cousin and her family had recently sold their home and were staying at her mom and dad's house. Her oldest son was confused and anxious. Every morning he'd wake up and ask; "Where am I?"

He was only used to living at his "old" house and disturbed about the change in bedroom, bed, and new routines. On top of all that change, he had a new brother to get used to. To help him accommodate, and because he was too young to do it himself, we surrogate tapped. I told my cousin to step behind his eyes and "be him" and tap about how he's feeling. She was spot-on with his confusion and negative thoughts. The changes in him were immediate and remarkable. He became calmer, relaxed and happier, even more cooperative.

I had her surrogate tap for her newborn son in the same way. She imagined how he felt and his reaction to her depression and anxiety energies. She noticed the positive changes in that baby right away! He started sleeping for longer periods of time and, like his big brother, was much calmer and relaxed.

From a physiological standpoint, hormonal swings are normal to re-balance the body postpartum. The less emotional stress in the past, the better the hormonal rebalancing experience. Whether PPD happens or not depends on the issues individual to each woman. That's what makes the difference.

It was such a gift for me to see my cousin with such an eagerness to try something new. Our work together cleared the path for even more change since then.

Cousin's transformation from weepy and overwhelmed to serene and balanced was miraculously quick! And it wasn't done with pills or conventional therapy. She didn't attend a support group and share scary mothering experiences. She used EFT.

Speaking of layers, remember my presentation with the "I dare you to crack my nut" soldiers at Fort Bliss? After that experience, I had another chance to breakthrough more "wounded warrior" barriers. This story has a very powerful and positive outcome.

CHAPTER FOURTEEN

Family War Zone

Anyone who has suffered traumatic events has "stress." Expanding the terminology of PTSD, all of my EFT clients have had some form of "post-traumatic stress." Obviously, at times faced with unimaginable horrors, military personnel have recently received the most attention. But it's not exclusively a military problem. As an EFT practitioner, I work with the effects of past traumas (PTSD) with just about every client.

Traumatic events cause an immediate disturbance in our energy system. The body downloads the trauma as in a cellular "jolt." This electrical shock ignites the sympathetic nervous system response. Without help with a release, this reflex will stay in the "on" position. It causes a chain of aberrant emotional reactions, disrupting inner peace or balance. As in postpartum depression, the severity of PTSD depends on the person's daily anxiety levels before the new events took place. This explains why some people are affected more than others. The more anxiety a person has, the less able they are to handle more of it. Over-load.

EFT rapidly and effectively helped one soldier and his wife: Nolan and Julia. They were already in the system for PTSD treatments at Fort Bliss, but without the results they had hoped for. Julia took the initiative to find a better solution for their problems, off base. She had heard about how EFT was being used to help war veterans. Without even knowing where to begin, she Googled "EFT El Paso" and found my name.

This initial step of seeking help outside the base is, in itself, empowering. By removing themselves from the "cattle herd mentality" (Nolan's own words), they took a proactive role in their own healing. Everyone has that choice. You can stay in one place and tread water, or you can find your own life preserver. In other words, "If what you're doing isn't working, try something else."

Nolan was a 35-year-old soldier, had been in the army for seven years and had three combat deployments. He had severe anxiety after returning from his third deployment to Iraq. Not long after he came home, Nolan checked himself into the William Beaumont Hospital. He had the feeling of wanting to "walk away from everything." With thoughts of going AWOL from the army and his own family, he felt like a failure. He rationalized they would be better off without him. He was admitted for "passive suicidal thoughts" and spent nine days in the hospital heavily medicated. He was being treated for insomnia, anxiety, and depression. They included art therapy to "express his emotions," all with no result. Nolan said that the anxiety medications "really, really freaked me out." The drugs seemed to intensify colors and lights. He also said he lived his daily life like he was still deployed, always on alert. He couldn't get close to or trust anyone, including his wife, and expected her to leave him eventually. All the while, the thought of yet another deployment was overwhelming.

When Nolan and Julia came to my office, they had viewed a YouTube EFT demonstration. But they never saw it used in person by an experienced practitioner. Nolan was quiet and unexpressive. After my grand EFT explanation, he sat through his first tapping round dead-panned. He told me it looked silly and was "just another bunch of crap." We addressed that belief next, because he simply told it as he saw it. It was strange looking and was different from anything he'd seen. It is also a very important component of a treatment to express any internal resistance. It's an important barrier that can stand in the way of deep healing.

After one tapping round of "this looks like a bunch of crap," he felt more relaxed. We laughed and got that out of the way. It definitely made it easier to get through his prepared list of specific events. I had asked, during the initial phone consult for him, to prepare a list of bothersome memories to work on. We took on the first big issue.

He had been having problems falling asleep and staying asleep for more than an hour at a time. Nolan informed me that he had run out of his sleep medications two days prior. I knew once we chiseled away at the big chunks, sleep would follow, so we did not tap directly on his sleep problem.

Some of his main issues were:

- The highest priority on his list was the recurrent image of his fellow soldier. He could see him lying dead with his brain hanging out of his skull.
- Because the next events happened over and over again, I asked for the first time, or the worst time it happened.
- The first time he had to kick in a door in Iraq. (He was a door kicker).
- The sound of the first mortar fly-over.
- The sight and sound of the first mortar hit. (Loud noises made him agitated and angry.)
- Anger about feeling used, following orders as a door kicker, and putting his life on the line. (Nobody cares). Note: see why later.
- The first visual memory of deplaning in Iraq, and the fear levels when he thinks of it now.

I thought it was a highly productive session. It ended with Nolan relaxed and feeling sleepy, a welcomed relief for him. For me, it was a good indication that the high priority issues resolved.

On their ride home from my office, his wife noticed that his demeanor had changed. His face looked completely relaxed, as if he had just returned from a well-needed vacation.

After we resolved his traumatic military events, childhood issues came to the forefront. He had unresolved past issues involving his mother. She was indifferent to him and unavailable. She walked away and abandoned her entire family, i.e., "she didn't care," just as the Army "didn't care" what happened to him. We addressed those issues at our second hour-long session. The best news was that working on the mother abandonment issues helped his marriage. The lack of trust in his wife came back to balance because the fear was gone.

After two sessions of EFT, Nolan feels he is completely over his PTSD. He also feels that his life overall has improved tremendously. In his own words, here is his progress report.

"The image of my fellow soldier killed in Iraq, the one I couldn't get out of my head, was completely gone after our first 10 minutes of EFT. It's been a couple of weeks since our first session, and if I do think of him now, it's when he was alive and healthy."

"I didn't like how I felt that the army used me being a door kicker; I was just following orders and putting my life out there. I've gotten over that anger as well."

"El Paso used to disturb me because some of the areas look like Iraq. But now, it's just El Paso, and we didn't even cover that in our session! That's what put me in the hospital in the first place, I was always on alert--because of the visual reminder."

"I was on sleep medications and having a real hard time going to sleep and staying asleep, even while I was hospitalized. I stopped taking the medications altogether, and now I'm sleeping the whole night every night. It's really great sleeping better. I handle stress a lot better now, and I don't need any of my medications. I feel calmer, and haven't had any anxiety problems since."

*Note: It's important you know that by law I cannot and do not advise any of my clients to stop their medications. I refer them to their medical doctors for tapering supervision.

Nolan and Julia attended our EFT Level 1 workshop shortly after his second session. Although she went there to support Nolan, Julia discovered the roots of her own issues. She discovered why Nolan's issues pressed so many buttons inside of her. One of them was the look on his face when he was heavily medicated. As a gift to all our attendees, we offered them a free half hour session. I did it as a gift and a jump-start on their own Storyboard Procedure list.

Having a close look at her husband's PTSD symptoms reminded Julia of the daily stress she endured as a child. Her mother was a heroin addict. The look on Nolan's face under the influence of his medications was exactly like her moms when she was high. Because Julia had a natural and resilient spirit, she was suppressing her past. It all seemed to work until the drugged face of her husband pushed an old button.

This is Julia's own testimonial after her half-hour private session.

"I now feel like I'm more "at one" with myself--more balanced, I don't feel so scattered. After the session, I went home and felt just like Nolan did when he left his first session. I could see how relaxed he was, and for me, everything was just slower, like life just slowed down. I felt more content, and for the very first time in my whole world, I was able to start and finish a task. At first, I was very reluctant to say anything to anyone because it almost seemed too quick and too good to be true! I was able to feel content, focus in on one thing at a time and finish it. And it happened again the very next day. By the third day, I was on the phone with my dad and telling him I had actually started and finished five different projects around my house, and it was a really good feeling."

"In my world, I consider myself a leader, and I can "fake it" by assigning other people on the teams that I'm on to make up for my weaknesses, so I don't appear so scattered. At home, my own family knows that I'm all over the place and for the first time ever, I know what balance feels like."

"Internally, I've always had quite a bit of anger, and I can say now, those levels are now down to about a 3, I might even say a 1 or a 2, and I feel very relaxed and excited for my day. Overall, I feel very relaxed. It's been great!"

"I've had really bad attention problems. I couldn't finish anything and felt scattered and always overwhelmed. When we were in the EFT class, I was able to see more clearly just how much discontent I've always felt. My attention problems were so bad that I could never sit down with my husband and watch a movie--but I watched one with him the other day--very unusual!"

"I have never been able to wake up my three kids after infant/toddler age. It's been a huge issue that I don't feel like I was ever aware of until my husband's PTSD showed up, and they started medicating him, which caused flashes of old memories seeing the drugged look on his face. Sleep faces remind me of my mother who was a heroin addict. My father who raised me was a pothead. I grew up hating sleep because it meant that I was alone and isolated."

"My oldest child is 13 years old, and I have never been able to go to her room and wake her up seeing her sleepy. Once my children got to that age I would yell at them from a distance, "It's time to wake up!" If I didn't get immediate responses from them, and if they weren't lined up like soldiers at the top of the stairs at attention, then I was irritated, mad, and then yell for having to wake them up myself. The hostility would surface, but I thought I was doing them a big favor by restraining my real anger. After my first session, I found the habit of standing at the top of the stairs to wake them was still there, but the anger is completely gone."

"Before my first session and after the EFT workshop, I went all the way up the stairs just to test it. It took more time for me to get mad. With each step I could feel it building internally, I thought, "I'm going to see the sleep face" and a few seconds later I could feel the hostility build. After my private session, I told myself I'm going up there again, I did it, and I was fine. I was able to have a conversation with my daughter and had a zero intensity of anger. I was absolutely able to stand there and look at her groggy face! My daughter and I look just like my mother, it was unbelievable that I was able to stand there and have a conversation with her while she was waking up. Its sad to me that I used to get angry at my own daughter. In ten years I have never been able to see her wake up! This is huge progress! The only thing remaining is for me to get rid of the weird habit of going to the edge of the stairs."

"I never realized I hated looking at my kids sleeping--who says that? After this all unraveled with EFT I realized that my problems were very deep--I was really running from my mom's sleeping face, I've been running for years."

Specific events we worked on:

I was afraid mom wouldn't wake up.
I was alone when she nodded off.
I felt betrayed each time she got high.
Mom didn't love me.
Mom didn't see me.
Sleep means lazy.

Nolan and Julia now have EFT as a tool to handle the normal, ongoing stresses of life. Using it regularly will continue to release long-held blocks to their happiness. They are part of a small but growing number of military PTSD victims who want a natural solution. They've taken the initiative to remove themselves from the conservative and ineffective approaches.

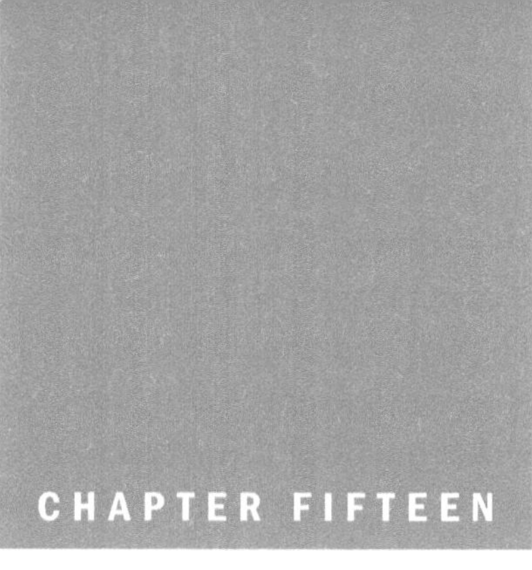

My "Groundhog's Day"

T he old guard has always resisted new approaches, and perhaps rightfully so. Since much that is "new" turns out to be of little use in the long run. Soldiers are in the unique position of placing themselves in wartime situations. You're expected to perform activities that are uncommon back in the states. They have the freedom to kill humans and destroy property without corporal punishment. It also gives the feeling of becoming "unleashed." Returning home, they're expected to go back to "normal" and function just like everyone else.

With over 20 years of a track record successfully treating stress-related conditions, EFT deserves more than a second look. It deserves to be recognized as a true "weapon" in the fight against PTSD. As essentially a self-help technique, it can be taught to soldiers and used in the field as needed. In the meantime, acceptance of this new type of treatment is slow, but the progress in treating PTSD conventionally is even slower. Even so, EFT will continue to forge ahead as a powerful treatment.

The Army already has "The Restoration and Resilience Center" on base at Fort Bliss for PTSD veterans. They're using relaxation therapies like Reiki, massage, with psychotherapy. I'm glad they were open to EFT; they will be again.

Our Fort Bliss experience was a wonderful learning opportunity and an honor for us. We're pleased the US Army gave a nod in the direction of Energy Psychology. I hope they do try again because it's highly effective. It's also cost-effective and it's a self-help tool every soldier can take with them anywhere. Knowing even the basics would save our armed forces a tremendous amount of suffering.

In my head, I reworked my whole Fort Bliss scenario. I was so pissed at myself, I went there first and tapped for anger. I used my "Bitch Tap Method™" (I'll tell you later) to get over it and move on. Oh, boy, did I bitch myself out over that one! Lol! I reached self-forgiveness, for trying too hard, and for under-thinking that whole presentation. As mom would say, it wasn't the end of the world.

I value my shoulda, coulda, woulda moments in life. I see them as opportunities for learning that help me modify, fine-tune, and step-up my game.

If I were in the movie "Groundhog's Day," the moment after the alarm went off, I would spring into action! And honey child, I'd serve them up some drama on a silver platter!

I would instruct the entire audience to gauge their current anxiety levels from 0-10. They would guess a number if they didn't think they had anxiety, and write it down. Next, I would lead one round of tapping for general anxiety, everyone following me. Okay, now what number is it? Write it down.

I would then proceed to work that entire room into one, great, big, giant, relaxation response. My parting shot is me turning on my heels and walking out of that room. Blowing out my tapping fingers like smoking guns, I'd whip em back into my imaginary holsters! (Think theme music of "The Good, The Bad, And The Ugly.") Sorry Mr. Eastwood, lol! Who-rah!

And we would bypass that horrific one on one with a soldier duel routine altogether. My audience would yawn, sigh, belch, feel relaxed, and feel lighter, together in the same room, at the same time. They could see the numbers of their intensities go down for themselves. There would be no denying a change. What a nice, non-scary introduction that would have been? I told you I learned from it! That entire experience, the good, the bad, and the ugly, served to help me to refine my approach to the advantage of EFT.

Bottom line, if I wanted to be the best I could be I had better start polishing my presentation! Now I'm confident I could work a stadium full of people, chew gum, and file my nails at the same time! I'm just saying.

Before I discovered the healing power of EFT, I was limping through life as an imposture. My acquired friends didn't really know me well, I shared very little, but I kept up appearances to the outside world. The rest of my highly driven professional life appeared to be fine, no evident cracks on the surface.

The old me had certain rules to live by. I made sure I had nothing but happy thoughts, listened to only happy, uplifting music, and no sad movies, ever. Hugs were good, just not too long of a hug, and only, ever, positive affirmations. That was my personalized elixir of positives, at least the ones I could control.

I still had plenty of negative childhood memories right at the forefront of my mind. I was able to recall any one of those bad memories chronologically, at any time, in great detail. Especially all alone with a few cocktails. Okay, maybe a few more.

Some people downplay the importance of negative childhood experiences. You should be able to "get over it" as the TV psychologist barbarically barks at his messed up subjects. Unfortunately, this popular declaration substantiates the old way of thinking before energy psychology.

When it comes to your health, on a cellular level, it's not that simple. Now studies support quite the opposite. Negative childhood experiences have everything to do with the adult that you become. It sets the stage how you accept information, and how you feel about yourself internally.

Believe me, I've interviewed enough clients to know that not everyone is ready to connect the dots. It's especially sad if they have a current problem that isn't working for them and want help. They'll say to me; "Childhood stuff doesn't bother me, I'm built different. I don't know why my siblings are so messed up, they should get over it, we had the same parents."

In my experience, negative childhood experiences stem from misinterpretations, miscommunications, and misunderstandings. Your age at the time of the negative event will determine the way you interpret it, and how deeply it lands. The tone and delivery of a negative message conveyed by a parent will determine how you accept it as your truth.

The misunderstanding about yourself, as a result, is before you realize how very little it had to do with "you." Instead, it's how much it had to do with the emotional state of the parent you had the problem with.

This is something I tell every one of my clients before we begin our work together. Working on core issues for many of us will include itemizing negative events with our parents. They're our main people, the mirrors through which we learn to see ourselves very early on. They weren't given any handbooks on how to raise us, given their background and their circumstances, they did the best they could at the time. We're not throwing stones at them, persecuting them, or playing the blame game. Not at all.

It's not my mission in life to change the mind of anyone who is unable to connect the emotional dots. It's my mission to shed light on the importance of the connection. Negative emotions always go hand in hand with serious health conditions and pain syndromes. In fact, their core issues are my forte'. You may have heard it many times, but I'll say it again. There is no separating the mind from the body, or the body from the mind.

For your own sake, and for the sake of your health, you have to be absolutely ready to look at everything and leave no stone unturned. In your own life experiences everything is important and impactful, and everything counts and matters. When it comes to you finally learning how to play on the same team instead of against yourself, the past is worth a second look.

The ACE Study, which we'll look at next, is strong supporting evidence that there is something to this. Of particular interest is something that has profound implications for health and wellness. It has been largely ignored by mainstream conventional medicine...it's too much to 'digest'...is the ACE study.

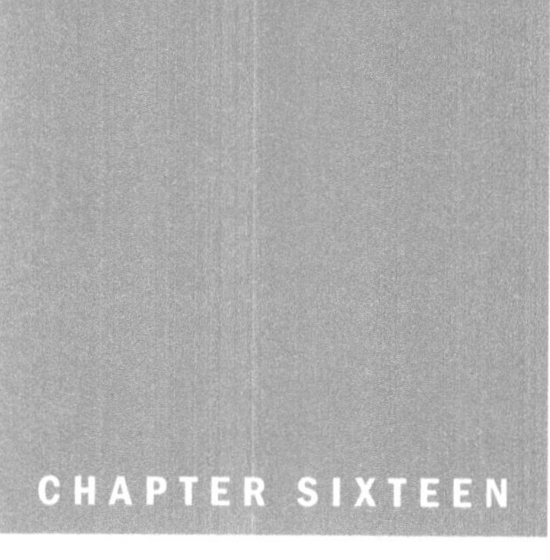

Trouble in Paradise

ACE stands for Adverse Childhood Experiences. The study was conducted by the CDC (Center for Disease Control and Prevention) and Kaiser Permanente. With over 17,000 participants in the study, surveys looked for instances of childhood abuse and trauma, specifically:

Physical abuse

Sexual abuse

Emotional abuse

Physical neglect

Emotional neglect

Battered parent

Household substance abuse (alcohol, drugs)

Mental illness

Parents separation or divorce

Household member arrested and jailed

It discovered that there is a direct correlation between toxic stresses in childhood, your adult health, and your lifespan.

"Moreover, the time factors in the study make it clear that time does not heal some of the adverse experiences we found so common in the childhoods of a large population of middle-aged, middle-class

Americans. One doesn't "just get over" some things." That's a quote from Vincent J Felitti, MD in his article on Adult Health and Adverse Childhood Experiences. [1] He then goes on to say "Clearly, we have shown that adverse childhood experiences are both common and destructive. This combination makes them one of the most important, if not the most important, determinants of the health and well-being..."

The majority of children in the study had at least one adverse experience while growing up. Having divorced parents, an alcoholic or drug addicted parent, and so forth. And, the effects add up when there is more than one category of toxic experience.

For example, having four ACE's was associated with a 700% increased likelihood of becoming an alcoholic. And twice as likely to develop cancer and four times as likely to develop emphysema.

And the stresses you experience can occur before you are even born, while still in the womb. Including stresses that your mother goes through while pregnant. Depression or partner violence have been shown to have epigenetic [2] effects on the baby as well.

The point here is that the negative impact of stresses during your childhood have a life-long effect on your health, on your lifespan.

It seems as if the negative energies continue to resonate within your body and mind, affecting the strength of your immune system. It affects psychological nurturing, the amount of nurturing you allow yourself emotionally and physically.

This will be covered in much greater detail in my next book, which will focus on mind-body renewal strategies. For now, here is a quick scan of the ACE Study on Wikipedia; and, Appendix V has more links to this important study.

(https://en.wikipedia.org/wiki/
Adverse Childhood Experiences Study)

I've included the ACE study to help you better understand the important role of negative childhood experiences, and how it pertains to you. ...and guess what? EFT is the quickest, easiest and most powerful self-help tool to get rid of that kind of stuff!

---

[1] https://www.academicpedsjnl.net/article/S1876-2859(09)00058-8/abstract

[2] https://www.whatisepigenetics.com/what-is-epigenetics/

Which is why on my website, EFTOne.com, I go to great lengths to explain how to use my Storyboard Procedure. With my unique template, you can use EFT to clear out your past in great detail. For the sake of inner peace and vibrant health, you're worth the time it takes.

So with that as context, here's more of my personal testimonial.

My dad was a US Navy veteran of both WW2, and later, the Korean War. As a Machinist's Mate Third Class, he was injured on board the destroyer, the US Theodore E. Chandler (DD-717). While loading a gun mount on rough seas, and firing, the shell casing flew backward hitting him in the head. Dad suffered a right-sided closed-head injury. He was unconscious for three weeks in a hospital in Japan. Hospitalized for six months altogether, and then was medically discharged. He came home deaf in one ear, and missing half a mouthful of teeth on the side of the injury.

Growing up in the early years, my big brother, Louie, and I, knew very little about our dad. We only knew he used to be in the Navy, he was a little hard of hearing, and he wore this thing in his mouth he called a partial.

Our life at home with dad was mostly hell, our house was never a happy home. There wasn't any room for happiness. Our house was full with the energy of his rage, and his horrible temper. Like navigating a minefield, we never knew when he would go off, and when he did, it was always devastating. If my brother or I were being punished, along with a brutal beating, we were also shunned. Sometimes we'd go a full week without him speaking to us. We weren't allowed to look at him while he was mad at us or sit at the same table for supper. He would tell us he "couldn't stand the sight of us." Our childhood was robbed by verbal abuse, hurtful name calling, and physical abuse. In the early 1960's, it went far beyond what was "acceptable" at the time, a spanking with a belt. I taught myself how not to cry because that would mean he won. I needed those victories to prove to him that no matter how hard he hit me or threw me, he could never break my spirit. He never did.

That was the reality of our secret life at home. Our trouble in paradise was a well-kept secret from our aunts, uncles, cousins, and family friends. That's because dad would magically turn into the nice, happy, funny guy when they came to visit our house. We loved having company over, it was always such a welcomed relief, it felt safe... at least temporarily. It was also nice to see mom and dad have fun and laugh. Their laughter would light up our entire house with such joy. It always made me feel like everything really was going to be okay, and it was until the company went home.

In my heart, I was always a prissy little girlie girl. I'd paint makeup on my dolls, and give them haircuts, all my Barbies had push-pin earrings. I loved to see my mom apply her makeup, wear her dangly jewelry, and wear pretty dresses. For play, I'd hook bobby pins together clipping them on my ears to make my own dangly earrings. I loved walking around the house wearing her big high heels. But as much as I yearned for it to be different, I was nobody's little princess. I took on a tomboy persona and wore clothes I could wrestle in and play tackle football with my brother. I had to prove to the neighborhood boys and everyone else how tough and strong I was.

Unfortunately for me, my parents hired a male teenage family friend as our babysitter. In front of us and the "babysitter" dad would threaten to "beat the hell out of" us if we misbehaved, or didn't do as we were told. That kid used dad's threat as leverage to demand I come downstairs from the bed, and "watch TV" (molested me). I was four years old.

I never told a soul about it for fear I did something wrong, and I would get punished. After he stopped "babysitting" us, I made it all go away, I never thought of it again. It felt like it never happened for years and years until later. As a small child in a traumatic event, our mind finds ways to compartmentalize them to survive. It's a good thing for us that our defense mechanisms for survival are very strong.

Louie, the focal point of dad's rage, could never do anything right. I was too young to recall when it first started, but for many years he wet his bed. Unfortunately for Louie, dad took it personally. The sound of his slow, heavy footsteps coming upstairs was my signal to hide in my closet and cover my ears. The terrible daily morning ritual of punishments varied from day to day. The crescendo of those led to a public humiliation event to "shame" him into stopping. And then we both had to go to school and try to act normal.

I can honestly say I couldn't have made it through those early grade school years without my one and only original crew of girls gathered around me to keep my mind off the trouble at home. Marcia, (my very first BFF since 4th grade) Tina, Jackie, and Vicky, we babysat, laughed, cried, shared our secrets, solved our troubles, and had epic sleepovers together. When I was allowed, spending the night at any one of their houses felt like a glorious vacation for me, a welcomed reprieve from the madness. To this day, through thick and thin, my old gang and I are still there for each other, that's the way it is. We still know and trust the original "us" and we still love each other fiercely...it's that tight.

I was too frightened for myself to ever help my brother. Mom, I know now, has suffered her entire life from anxiety and panic attacks. During the violence, she would retreat to another room and tread lightly until it all cooled down. I explored this issue further while working with a critically ill client. A Gestalt psychotherapist with father issues, his professional specialty was anger management for men.

The Major Blind Spot

Negative emotions beneath serious diseases and pain syndromes are my EFT specialty. There are exceptions to the rule, but I end up working almost exclusively on anger issues. I found some very consistent observations and reactions from clients. It's a "hidden aspect," that when uncovered often causes profound shifts and insights. I've come to call it the Good Parent/Bad Parent conflict.

This insight is commonly overlooked by those who were abused and mistreated by a parent. The "bad" parent is easily the source of many tapping issues. Their misdeeds provide an obvious source for many specific negative events. Meanwhile, the parent who was "good" was typically the island in the storm of the household. The reality is, the "good parent" is key, and a major core issue, a "blind spot." Uncovering this realization leads to deeper, more thorough emotional healing. This leaves no stone unturned.

The bottom line is one parent was abusive, and the other parent let it happen and didn't protect you. The good parent may even be responsible for setting up that whole dynamic for their own reasons. More about that later.

What I mean by that is this: typically the client is focused on the obvious "mean" parent, and canonizes the other. But I consistently find the "sainted parent" to be the real source of rage. This surprising discovery is almost always unapparent to the client. It's an outlook that refocuses the source of rage and raises new abandonment issues to address. Introducing this different view to the client doesn't go without resistance. We examine the "possibility" of the good parent being an issue when I see it is necessary.

A good parent is definitely a touchy subject, and there are variables in every situation. But there is an underlying sense of guilt in seeing them in a different way, "How could I say that when she/he was so good to me?"

My ideal clients have the motivation to get better, and they are open to exploring whatever it takes. You especially owe it to yourself to do that if your health is at stake. The less ideal clients are those who are only in love with the "quest" to get better. It makes them feel proactive and in control to seek help, but they aren't willing to do the work. That's the problem. They have secondary gains being sick, it gets them something they need (love). I can see that in a hurry, and it's not up to me to take that away from them. It's up to them to see it isn't working for them first. The path to self-help and healing is very deep and personal. I have respect for everyone, even if I can't work with them as a client.

During sessions, my approach is to coax the client into "trying on" different feelings. This is the time a good pre-frame is useful for assuring them that there is no disrespect intended. As Gary Craig called it, "garbage and gold." It's an intuitive guess or a hunch for a setup phrase that will either land or not, with no harm done, and no harm intended. Some "guesses" can be garbage, but some can be gold, hitting the issue right on point.

When it comes to the topic of parents, let me emphasize that we are not trying to play the "blame game" here and leave it at that. It's to re-distribute the anger and put it into the proper perspective as an adult. Not the way you, as a child, interpreted your parents. That's when you're stuck, and those are the thoughts that keep you in pain. It's a relief to the client to realize that it takes one passive parent to allow the aggressive one to call the shots.

The ultimate goal here is to achieve clarity, forgiveness and deep healing. So it is important to reach a place of understanding about both parents. Personal peace falls somewhere in the middle of all this.

There is a multitude of reasons why one parent is willing to stay in an abusive situation with children. With regard to the good parent, it's important to recognize that powerlessness is a core issue.

I wrote this article because, while working with this client, I had a pivotal discovery about another of my own blind spots. It's unprofessional to make a session be about me and not the client, so I never told him about it. But our subconscious parallels uncovered a new aspect of my life by proxy. I'm very grateful for that. Here's the story.

William is well-respected, and a world-renowned Gestalt psychotherapist for over 40 years. Interestingly enough, he's an expert in his field, specializing in men's anger issues. He's famous for his anger management workshops for men. It's his life's work, and he loves helping men find their voice, and own their issues. He provided a safe place for them to express themselves in his workshops.

He called me because he was suffering from pancreatic cancer and I had a pretty good track record with it. He found my "Angry Pancreas" article on the internet. His doctors told him to get his affairs in order, he was on his way out sooner than later. Based on his traditional, professional training and educational background, he was skeptical about EFT. But, like so many of my seriously ill clients, desperation led him to at least try it.

William, the youngest of two sons, came from an affluent family. His father was in a political position of great prestige and authority. Unfortunately for the family, he was also an alcoholic. In this case, his mother, the "Saint," had to keep up appearances as the perfect wife and mother in public. But in privacy, she accommodated an aggressive and dominating alcoholic husband. Above all else, she was a genteel Southern lady who never acted out inappropriately.

The mother had a long history of bouts of depression and withdrawal. Without warning, she would take to her bed for weeks at a time. William understood this intellectually and had nothing but compassion for all she endured. As for William, anger was a very bad thing to express. In fact, the only way he could express his own rage years later was to be intoxicated just like, guess who?

By Williams own admission, he worked on his issues with some of the top psychotherapists in his field. He spent years sorting out his past to heal and enhance his understanding of himself, and his clients.

At our initial interview, he told me his father had been "the bane of his childhood existence." Father was the topic of his many years of

Cognitive Behavioral Therapy (CBT). He assured me that after all that work there was nothing left to deal with about his father. He suggested we should look at other aspects of his adult life he felt were undone.

Throughout his personal and professional life, he regarded himself as "very easy going." William, an accomplished intellect in his field, set an example of how to control anger, and rise above it.

Even after a very painful divorce (unfaithful wife), he gamely took it on the chin. Instead of confronting him, he shook hands with his "best friend," the man she left him for, and let bygones be bygones. Without argument or need of explanation, he bid his wife farewell after 20 years of marriage. He was proud of how civilized he had been. Besides, he'd be just like his father if he did display anger, if he looked or acted as if he had fallen apart. It would prove that he really didn't have it all together. God forbid he act angry, that would mean he wasn't evolved. His reputation at stake, he had to keep up appearances.

CHAPTER EIGHTEEN

Rage? What Rage?

Our first session involved coaxing an anger response at his "best friend," who had an affair with his wife. I used my "Bitch Tap Method™", which elicited a true rage response and shock at his own reaction. The result of that session was a cessation of the constant 8-9 intensity level of pain he felt in his mid-back, a knife-like stabbing pain (get the metaphor on this one?). That got his attention, and he decided that there really was something to this "energy stuff."

Talking about his father's drunken rages, I asked William where his mother was in all this? He said, "that's a good question, but let's have a look." He told me his mother always wanted everything to be perfect, including him. She was always fidgeting with his hair, his collar, constantly "fixing" him. She insisted he always look presentable because, according to William, appearances were everything. "That's just the way mom was, everything was always wrong for her. Nothing was ever good enough or right." With that, I suggested, for exploratory purposes, that we do a round of tapping about that. I wanted to see if there was any emotional charge about having to look perfect. He replied, "OK, if you think so, but I doubt it."

"I can accept myself even though mom wasn't satisfied with the way I looked."

After a round of tapping, William said he felt some anger welling up in his chest. And what started at a zero emotional charge, spiked up to a 7 level of intensity. It made him feel like something was wrong with him because she was obvious about her disapproval; either rearranging his hair in front of others, or commenting that his attire wasn't right.

Then, an old memory came up about her sending him back to his room to change his clothing. This was after he had taken great care trying to look his best for a birthday party. He felt sad and mad at the same time about this event. Following his lead, we continued.

"Even though my best wasn't good enough that day, something is wrong with me, maybe I can accept myself."

He got even angrier after two rounds of "there's something wrong with me." It went up to a 10 level intensity. He said; "You know Rossanna, to this day I refuse to wear a coat and tie, God damn it!"

Other tapping phrases followed:

"Even though mom wasn't perfect she expected me to be."

"Even though I always wish mom was like Billy's mom."

"Even though I don't know why she even had us if she was so sick, to begin with."

"Even though I was born to make her happy, and it didn't work."

"Even though I could never make her happy."

"Even though I never knew when she would get sick again and leave us alone with dad."

An intuitive thought popped up suddenly that prompted an extended setup phrase. We had much to do yet, and with this new can of worms opened, I thought we could fit in clarity and forgiveness. It was worth a shot.

"Even though mom felt wrong inside, everything was wrong for mom, and she tried her best to make me right, but it made me feel wrong; I can accept how I feel about this now, and choose clarity, so I can fully forgive her."

Reminder phrase: "It was the way mom felt about herself; it was never about me; my appearance was the only thing she could control; she could allow herself to feel better when I looked just right, knowing what I know now, I can feel compassion for her inner struggle and forgive her with all my heart."

William was very surprised that this small issue with his mother, who could do no wrong, had turned to such anger. That's the beauty of EFT; if it's wafting around on a cellular level, it will surface with tapping! After testing and retesting this issue, he felt it was a zero.

But it gets better!

The next unexpected negative event with his mom was a "wait until your father gets home" issue. This specific issue was a memory he said he had spent many hours on in therapy, the focus being on his father only. Even so, here it was again, with his mother being the focus this time.

His mom knew the ferocity of her husband's temper fueled by drinking on his way home from work. But she consistently assigned him the task of disciplining the children. William recalled being very young (2 or 3 years old) when this happened. He couldn't remember why his oldest brother got into trouble. But he recalled waiting with him in the bedroom until his father got home. There was an obviously high emotional charge in just saying that much out loud. So I approached the event by sneaking up on it using therapeutic dissociation. It's called the "Tearless Trauma Technique." We tested his intensity levels and tapped until it was low enough to comfortably tell the story.

"Even though I was afraid he would kill you."

"Even though I can still see him chase you around the table."

"Even though I can still see myself crying in the closet."

"Even though I didn't think he would ever stop beating you."

"Even though I was too small to help you."

"Even though I was too afraid to help you."

I asked him where his mom was during all this? He said, "Standing there watching it happen."

"Even though you (mom) didn't stop it."

"Even though you knew what would happen and set him up anyway."

"Even though you didn't give a damn."

"Even though I #%&*ing hate you for that."

"Even though you're a coward."

"Even though I can't trust you."

William was stunned at his anger toward her after our session. Perhaps there were reasons why his dad was so angry and couldn't cope? Could it be possible that dad felt he needed to be anesthetized (have drinks) just to come home to his own reality? Why did he punish his dad by rebelling and embarrassing him for so long? Were his actions the misinterpretations of a child who couldn't understand adult problems? Maybe dad wasn't such a bad guy after all?

He came to the realization that his mother actually had anger by proxy. Her southern upbringing dictated it's not genteel or lady-like to act "ugly." Her stuffed down emotions were likely core issues behind her depressions. She, the passive parent set up angry responses for the aggressive parent, her husband. She wasn't there for either of her children in the biggest way. She either coped by escaping into her closed-bedroom-door depression or orchestrated rage-filled punishments. With everyone being her pawn, it was easier for her to "witness" anger, allowing her husband to do it for her. She stood by and passively watched without stopping the brutality.

William came to realize that her passive aggression was extreme. "If she had had the courage and clarity to love and respect herself, to protect herself and her children, none of this would have happened." There is truth to that; the family dynamics would have been very different. Meanwhile, other insightful "mother" epiphanies resonated with him for the rest of the week. He used them as material for his homework between our sessions. He was my most compliant client in that respect.

I received an email from William a day after his "good parent" session. To me, it was living proof of how very profound his inner healing had been, that he really "got it" and acknowledged it. A man with his background could have had real professional resistance issues. [3] But we had already addressed that possibility early on. He wrote me an email.

"After working on this issue on Wednesday, I had a sudden thundering realization that I did learn about forgiveness, and I learned it from my father, but missed the lesson because I was so anti-anything-father. And I remember well, on a cellular level, the feeling of utter relief and freedom and joy at being forgiven, which comes back to me now in a physical sensation of elation. I made a list of all the people I had ever harmed or who had harmed me, and I've been tapping and struggling to forgive them and me. From inside my mother's world,

---

[3] See my article exploring the issue of professionals resisting getting help from others https://www.dropbox.com/s/3bcnxu32aximq4h/Professional%20Resistance.pdf?dl=0

this wasn't going very well and seemed to have no end, and now, from inside my father's world, which is now very much my own, forgiveness comes so easily, with the grace of a summer breeze, that I am in a state of amazement and tears."

William would eventually succumb to his illness. There comes a time when the body is beyond the point of regaining homeostasis. The physical body is too far gone and incapable of catching up.

Codependent Comedian

The value of EFT, used as an "emotional hospice" before the transition to death, is priceless. Resolving past emotional issues is the ultimate cleanse. And it's a true confession of the heart. Cleaning up the unfinished business in your life can only promote deep inner peace. The emotional comfort is soothing and heals the heart. I still view my experience with William as a great success for him in the grander scheme. His entire professional career centered on men's anger issues. That's because they related to his own anger issues. The very emotion he so honestly and diligently sought to be rid of his entire life, went away forever with EFT. Reconciliation and forgiveness lightened the scales for his passing considerably. Rest in peace William, bravo to you, and your work, and a life well lived.

Meanwhile, back to growing up at our house. When it came to his temper, dad never considered our holidays sacred or special. But it was the one thing mom, Louie, and I enjoyed together the most. We'd decorate the entire house, bake cookies, dye eggs, and wrap presents, and play holiday music. We were always excited and filled with the holiday spirit for whatever the occasion. And that's what made it so unbelievably sad and disappointing when dad would focus his rage on mom or one of us. Once he got started, he couldn't stop being angry or reason with any of us. With no chance for resolution or apologies, it would ruin the entire day until we went to bed. Christmas, Easter, a birthday, no big deal. There was no escaping the little white house that rage built.

I used to beg my mom to leave him, but she never could, she could never stand up to him either. I was too young to understand it at the time, but her reality was, she was a stay at home mom with four children. And she's Catholic, Latin Catholic, uber Catholic.

As a side note, stemming from the aftermath, I was a little bit codependent, to say the least. I was angry from years of witnessing mom's disrespect and mistreatment. Especially after all she did to try and please him, I was profoundly pissed off. Not only from what Louie and I went through, I was angry for her too, by proxy. If she couldn't defend herself, I was strong enough for both of us. Gulp. I took on the role of her defender. Being her avenging angel kept me enmeshed in needless family drama many times over the years. Righting all wrongs for her (my choice entirely, not hers) was an exhausting, full-time job.

I stopped it once I recognized the toll it took on me emotionally and psychically. Whew! Glad that's over! Eventually, I taught mom how to stop a panic attack without getting into all the core issues. EFT has always been successful at stopping her panic attacks right in the moment. Since then those episodes have been fewer and far between. I've also shown her how to tap for fear and anxiety, to be less fearful about speaking her truth. I continue to help her (when she asks) feel more entitled to her feelings.

My codependency was an issue for my EFT self-work. Eventually, I was able to resign from my self-appointed position as her defender. I discovered that aside from offering her some amount of comfort, it never "fixed" anything for her. I actually made things worse by enabling her to remain disempowered. My rescuing super-hero act (okay, Wonder Woman) did not allow room for her own growth. Nor was I providing opportunities for her to practice setting her own boundaries. I can tell you this, through my EFT self-work, my boundaries remain intact.

As a kid, I got good at navigating dad's mood swings through trial and error. I practiced my comedic timing by saying something funny before things escalated. I taught myself how to imitate character voices on TV, a skill now well-honed. I mastered the Elly May Clampett accent (the daughter from The Beverly Hillbillies) and called him "paw" instead of dad. With that voice, I was able to sass-back my own daddy whenever I could get away with it. It used to make my parents laugh, and I sounded so silly, but I didn't care; it lightened things up in a hurry. The most important thing was I got to say what I meant to say to him cloaked in humor without getting killed.

Through the alchemy of love and food, my mother was an accomplished cook. And she could majorly throw down in her own kitchen. I'm serious when I say everyone wanted to eat at our house. She wowed our relatives with her creations at family gatherings. She was never afraid to experiment with exotic dishes from her many cookbooks. Before dad came home from work, we would grocery store hop to seek out the finest ingredients. Supper was presented promptly at 5:30.

Mom's vast repertoire of meals came from a combination of old family recipes and her own ingenuity. By taste and memory she replicated the dishes from her mother, the original kitchen rock star. I can still remember every sumptuous meal she ever made, especially Sunday dinners.

Dad's parents, Sito, (grandmother) and Jido, (grandfather) were immigrants from Latakia, Syria. Remembered for her shyness, and her ability to save money, my Sito could cook. She would wake up at the crack of dawn to make Syrian bread every morning for her family of 11 children and her husband. After losing two infant sons to illness, she spoiled my dad. Dad had his favorite meals he remembered the best, and mom made sure he ate them.

To please dad, and "make him happy," mom made it her business to master the art of Arabic cooking. She did this, of course, her way, by stepping it up with her own spices and adding garlic to the foods she deemed bland. Mom learned from the masters. She collected recipe variations and specialties from the little old Maronite Catholic church [4]ladies. She also received special tutorials from dad's sisters who learned from their mom.

Mom's food was our sustenance, but more than that, it was our protective shield. Night after night she would weave our little, broken family back together again at our supper table. Her gift was bountiful servings of love and comfort, from her to us. If her piano music could calm the savage beast, so could her cooking. I always appreciated that

---

[4] Maronite Catholics see here: http://www.cnewa.org/default.aspx?ID=56&page typeID=9&sitecode=hq&pageno=1

show of love from her very much. Very early on, even though she could never say it, I got the message.

From the time I was old enough to understand, mom stated the importance of being a woman with a college degree. She'd say, "A pretty face is a dime a dozen, get an education, find a career, get out of here or you'll never get anywhere. Don't be afraid to go out into the world experience life. You have the power to be anything you want to, so always think big, and reach for the sky." It was our truth, our mother-daughter secret girl-power mantra I never doubted, not once. I had my mom's stamp of approval. Although I was going to miss her terribly, I was leaving when the time came, and that was that.

Consequently, my feet never firmly planted in the green, green grass of my Indiana home. I would never take root there, rather, it would be my launch pad. Years later as a Flight Attendant, mom's dad, "graham-paw," (in my Elly May voice) told me that I traveled around like a Gypsy without a home. He was correct, and it was exactly how I liked it.

Up until the time I graduated from high school, my life, as I saw it, was in waiting. It was a countdown until I turned 18 when I could leave without dad stopping me. With mom's encouragement, secretly, I applied for college. On my own, I borrowed a friend's car and drove myself to East Chicago to apply for grants to finance my education. The time came when I had to ask dad for help filling out his financial statement to help me qualify for a school loan. Dad told me; "Who do you think you are? What makes you think you can go to college? I'm not sending you anywhere, you don't belong there, I'm not filling out anything! It's none of their damn business how much money I make!" But that only fueled my determination, I found another way. I anxiously awaited to hear by mail either my college acceptance or denial.

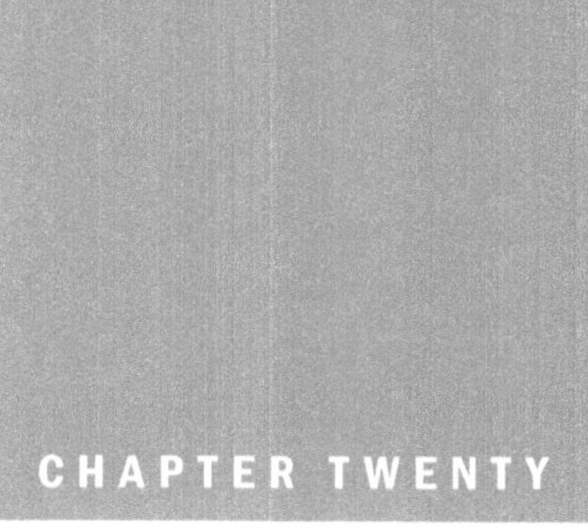

She's Leaving Home

I finally received my scantron registration card from Indiana University, Bloomington. But dad saw it first and opened it. He confronted me, held it up to my face, and ripped it up throwing it on the floor. I dropped to my hands and knees picking up all the little pieces. Stuffing them into an envelope, I said a silent prayer hoping they'd still accept me. Because now, my college entrance card was destroyed.

The day I left, dad said to me, you think you're big enough to leave home? Don't you ever ask me for a dime! As I headed toward the door to leave, he said, "You aren't going anywhere." I spun around and looked at him straight in the eyes and said, "Watch me." I hitched a ride with a friend, leaving my mom waving goodbye on the steps outside the front door. I couldn't even think about what she was going to go through with him after I left. That time, I chose me. I was 17 years old.

One of the many reasons why I picked Indiana University in Bloomington, was because it's a Big Ten college. That meant it was a well-respected institution, and I was proud to attend. It gave me credibility, and that helped my self-esteem; well okay, my boyfriend was there too. The best thing was, it's on the opposite end of the state from my hometown, (4 hours to be exact) and I'd be free to do what I want! Whoop! Whoop!

Ugh, I was shocked by how homesick I felt those first few weeks, but I really was. It felt like a dull heartache in my chest. The whole contrast was a drastic shift from the volatile, and unpredictable. From that to a non-drama existence on my own in a dormitory full of noisy strangers. I missed my mama. I met some really nice girls on the 6th floor of Willkie Quadrangle, they came from all over the United States. We had a blast with all the new activities at school. It began with the Little 500 tricycle race, we even made up a song about us 6th-floor girls in the name of school spirit! And in the name of common decency, I won't repeat it! Lol! Let's chalk it up as kooky college schoolgirl hijinks!

Then came "Rush." When the time came to pledge a sorority, I knew nothing about it except that it must be an exclusive rich girl's club. Only rich girls need apply. I immediately counted myself out. You had to have nice clothes, a car, and lots of money. I saw how excited everyone was, especially the legacy girls who were accepted into the house that they wanted. Figuring if you can't join them, beat them, I decided it was time for me to live like an independent big girl. I'd do it without some "housemother" breathing down my neck, and worse, a curfew. I was in for one of the best times of my life.

While on campus I ran into a hometown girl who graduated from high school with my big brother, Louie. She was a beautiful, raven-haired, spirited, Lebanese girl. The best thing was, she had a wonderful sense of herself, a great personality. Her name was Susan. She wanted to rent a house and was looking for a roommate, it was perfect timing. We rented a stinky, old, one bedroom house on Cottage Grove Avenue.

As much as we cleaned and scrubbed that place, we could never get the smell of stale grease out of our little kitchen. Getting to know each other was easy, and I didn't realize it at the time, but she and I were perfectly suited. We were meant to be together because she would be the pivotal person in my life who introduced me to the feeling of Arabic pride. I channeled my "inner Syrian" through the food we made together, the music, and the graceful movement through dance. Thus began the process of reconnecting and finding common ground with dad... eventually.

Her parents were divorced, and she was raised without a father in the house. I, on the other hand, had a dad, and as much as I hated it, he stayed and made us miserable. Susan never liked hearing me complain about dad. She'd always find a way to defend him, saying how I was lucky to have one (eye roll). I didn't want to hear that, I wanted an ally on all fronts. I did stop complaining about him though, I wasn't getting anywhere with her anyway. I never argued the point, because I saw her point, and more than anything, I respected her.

Very feminine and lady-like herself, Susan taught me refinement. By example, she showed me how to be more of a lady, and shook the tomboy out of my personality. I took copious notes, believe me, she was an awesome role model.

Her own mother was very dignified and refined; in fact, I loved her whole family. They all felt like family to me, including her very strong, stern, serious, and hilarious Sito (grandmother). Since my Sito died way before I was born, I adopted her as my own. She was my ideal of what a Sito should be; loved, feared and respected.

To me, Susan remains to be one of the best Middle Eastern dancers I've ever seen. Our nights were spent ordering pizzas (our favorite treat) and studying for a bit. We'd take our breaks by throwing on a Mohammed El-Bakker album and freestyle dance to the music of "Port Said." With our Arabic power music, we shook our teezna (butts) and shimmied our shoulders, (God, I tried). I practiced waving my hands gracefully like hers, as we danced from one end of the house to the other. I treasure those times together, and thanks to her, I still dance to the same music around the house with my dogs! It's hilarious to see them hopping and jumping alongside me. Smile. And it totally gives me an edge in Zumba class too! Lol!

We both had a crush on Al Pacino, we were in love with him. For her it was the "Frank Serpico" character, for me, it was "Michael" from "The Godfather." We would say; "smallah" in Arabic (when someone is very good looking) every time we talked about him. We kept a poster of his face in our bathroom, even kissing it occasionally lol! Okay, we were still teenagers! One night we even tried placing a phone call directly to him in NYC. We weren't successful, (I bet he's glad) but together, we were bold. We had so much fun, we never once had a disagreement.

The two of us glamor-pusses took the campus library by storm to "study," but in reality it was THE place to see and be seen. We created cute outfits between her clothes and mine to make that scene. With kohl-lined eyes, and "Mocha Meringue" lipstick, we were sultry Middle Eastern fabulous.

At night we were always safe together in our little house. We ate well, laughed, danced, and studied...and healed. Our cultural dance was an important component in the awakening of our Root Chakra. The deep connection between ourselves and the earth between our toes was set into motion.

Susan taught me all the big sister things I wanted/needed to know about men and life. She read poems by Kahil Gibran and taught me about ancient Middle Eastern history. Even though I still can't string more than a few words together, I also learned a little bit of Arabic from her. For the first time in my entire young life, and after such a disconnect with my dad, I was beginning to feel my own roots. And for once, I liked it.

I lasted there for almost two years, but I never really felt like I belonged in college, more like an imposter. Who was I was kidding? I wasn't good enough to be there anyway, and besides, who did I think I was? I had no business being there, I'm not very bright, I'm stupid, I'm just a dumbass. It wasn't a hard decision for me to drop out of school when I finally made the decision to walk away. Besides, my boyfriend just graduated and was leaving, and who would I be without him? Yeesh. Even though she tried to talk me out of it for my own good, I was sad to leave Susan. She remains to be my soul sister, and I have nothing but love, respect, and gratitude for her. I always remember her for all the ways she touched my life. Shukran Susan, wallah.

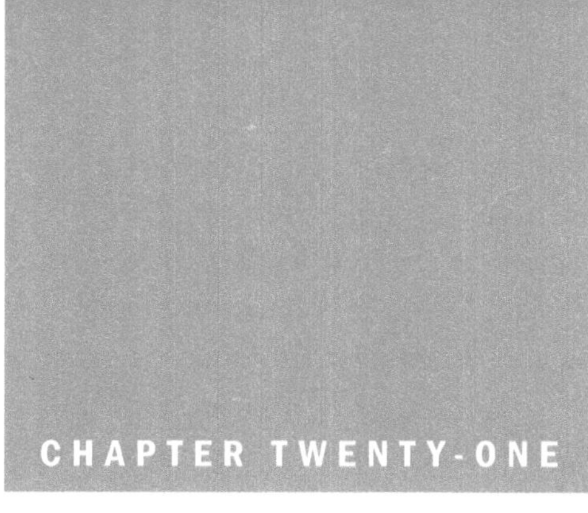

Sky Goddess

Per my mom's advice to leave and go "bigger," (go big and don't go home) in 1977, I set a goal to become a Flight Attendant. I'll never forget how I blew my interview with Continental Airlines. I bought myself a black suit for the occasion from the clothing store I worked at back home, at the Marquette Mall.

Continental flew me to Los Angeles from Chicago for my interview. I was driven in a company vehicle to their Inflight Services offices off-site near the LAX airport. When I was told to wait and be seated by the glamorous receptionist, I started to get scared. I learned I would be interviewing with a vice president. Yikes!

I can only describe it as me having an out of the body experience, but when I walked through the door to meet the VP, I clammed up, and couldn't say a word. There he sat behind a huge desk, in a big chair, looking very professional and intimidating. He stared down his nose at me, took stock, and asked me a few questions. I choked the answers out of my mouth and sat frozen. He jotted down a few notes in a file, looked up and me and said; "Thank you for coming, Rossanna, it was nice to meet you. The receptionist will show you where to meet the car back to the airport."

I was officially dismissed, given the bum's rush: Beat it kid, this ain't for you, bah-bye! I stood waiting for the car in disbelief that the whole thing was over so fast, after all the excitement leading up to this very moment. This was it for me.

With the sounds of airplane engines in the background, and the smell of jet fuel wafting around, I told myself off. "This is your one big moment and you blew it, stupid! You've spent your entire childhood with your head inside the lion's mouth, but you're afraid of this little guy? Turn around and march right back in his office and tell him who you are!"

And that's exactly what I did next. I brushed passed the receptionist saying "I forgot something," and walked through his door without knocking. With a surprised look on his face, I walked up to his desk, shook his hand, and reintroduced myself. "I came back because I didn't express myself the way I wanted to," I told him. "Give me a few more minutes of your time, and I'll tell you why I'm right for this position." When I saw him smile and listen, even chuckle, I knew I had made my impression. When I finished, he thanked me again and said I would hear from them in two weeks. I flew back to Chicago quite satisfied...I didn't know how I did that, I didn't know I had it in me! I had just discovered I had a nice sized set of huevos! Apparently, momma taught me very well....so had dad.

When my acceptance letter came in the mail, I opened it and read it wide-eyed in disbelief. Clasping it to my chest, I sank to my knees and screamed out loud with pure joy, tears streaming down my face! Continental's Flight Attendant scrutiny was so notorious, so picky, I couldn't believe I made it! This would be my very first major victory. I was the girl who's best friend got picked over her for cheerleading squad more than once, the one who never got asked to prom...both of them. Things were going to be different now. Working for a major airline brought with it a whole new meaning of acceptance for me. It was a personal game changer that automatically increased my levels of self-worthiness! It also elevated my self-respect from down to up (or so I thought). It was a huge event for me. Thank you, God, I needed that! The job title of Flight Attendant meant instant credibility from the general public. Scrutinized by the best in the airline industry, instant integrity was a bonus. Small town girl makes good, I was off to see the world.

I was only 19 years old when they hired me, the second youngest in our Flight Attendant graduation class. I made an absolutely wonderful living for being so young. They gave us makeovers, taught us manners, diction, how to walk, how to speak to celebrities, and most importantly, emergency procedures, how to evacuate an airplane under any circumstance. I worked with many beautiful, colorful, and absolutely hilarious Flight Attendants. Before I was senior enough to bid my own schedule, being on standby, I had a constant mix of coworkers. Since we all had similar personality traits, there was rarely, if any, inflight drama. For ten years total, in 3-inch heels, I sashayed my way across the skies. My sky sisters and I sassed, served, and potentially saved hundreds of thousands of passengers along the way.

I'm so grateful to still have some of my wonderful friends from that time, Susie, Dona, Tom, and Cathy (Cay-Cay). Thanks to Facebook, more have resurfaced into my life, and I'm still looking for those I miss. I loved all of my sky sisters, male and female. It turns out, they were my true college sorority.

A cousin of mine who I hadn't seen for years, Mona, hired on as a Flight Attendant for Continental. Her mom called my mom (they're sisters) and arranged for her to stay with me until she got settled. It was her first time living away from home, and ages since we'd seen last seen each other. We didn't know if we would recognize each other at first. All dolled up, (of course) I pulled up to the curb at Houston airport in my shiny little black Porsche 911. I rolled down my window, she walked up to the car and asked; "Are you my cousin? I thought you were older!" I replied, "Hop in kid, you're in for a ride!" It was so sweet, because she didn't know what to expect, and now she did. After many hilarious and wonderful shopping excursions together, we became the closest of friends. "Always buy quality," she said.

Even though I was senior to her new-hire standby schedule, we managed to fly together. We enjoyed our layovers, face masks and gym time, comparing mothers and fathers. Through her, I was able to see my mom better by contrast, and better understand her Mexican culture. We got to know each other very, very well. She helped to reinforce self-nurturing skills which I'm grateful for. I still adhere to them today like setting aside extra "me" time for self-care. In the precious time we spent together in the kitchen, she dazzled me with her culinary artistry.

My cousin was the first of my bazillion cousins who didn't think I was off on some weird tangent (judge me) because of EFT. Instead, she was the first to learn it.

Like an aunt of ours, Mona was born with the natural propensity for salesmanship. She's good at it, and she sells skin care as a dual career. She learned how to use EFT to improve the quality of her sales skills. She knows how to break sales barriers, sharpen her focus, and release dread for sales calls. Her loyal and loving friendship remains a very important part of my life. I call her "Cousin Dearest."

As a Flight Attendant for a major airline, I loved meeting people from all walks of life. I met presidents, sports figures, rock stars, musicians, famous singers, and famous actors. I loved learning about different people, cultures, customs, and languages. The Flight Attendant lifestyle was such an advantage for a small town kid like me. I was able to see so many different cities and eat at fabulous restaurants in exotic locations. We were always invited to the hottest, most exclusive disco clubs, so I had fun everywhere we flew. I enjoyed the best beaches and toured all the sights throughout the South Pacific with fellow crew members on long layovers. But my personal life was very lonely and very isolated.

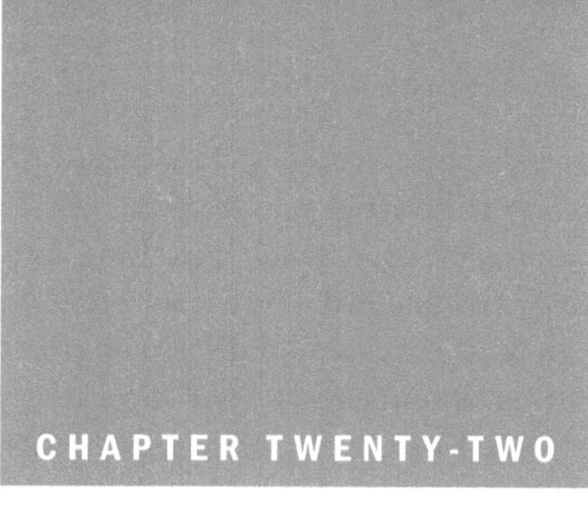

Not So Goddess-y

In the 70's we looked more like "Barbies" although we preferred "Sky Goddess" lol! We worked our flights in full makeup, big hair, fitted uniforms, manicured nails, false eyelashes, and three-inch heels. We looked glamorous, and being a Fight Attendant was considered a glamorous career. But it was only a facade for public mystique. Continental Airlines advertising catchphrase was "The Proud Bird With The Golden Tail." In reality, the truth known, we worked our ever-loving, golden tails off!

Most of my female coworkers were very beautiful women and some past Miss USA contestants. I struggled with body image. As my own worst critic, I put myself down because I was never happy with the way I looked. I hated certain body parts (from my feet up) I felt were "ugly."

Comparing myself to gorgeous coworkers made me feel like I didn't fit in; in reality, thinking those negative thoughts, I was making damn sure I didn't. I wasn't good enough to be there either. A part of me felt like I didn't belong with these people. Besides, who did I think I was anyway?

The other thing going against me back then was my financial life or lack thereof. Growing up in the late 60's the unspoken rule for most of us girls out of high school was to get married and be taken care of. No need wasting money on college if you're going to be a stay at home mom. For me, seeing what the marriage thing looked like up close growing up, that was the last thing I ever wanted. It was the tail end of the "Mad Men" mentality back then, especially in a small town.

So, I had zero experience in money management. And ill-equipped for financial planning to invest in a place of my own. I made very good money and blew it on rent, trips, jewelry, clothing, and sports cars, you know, the essentials. I had no real money savvy peers or a single person I could go to for guidance because I didn't know who to trust.

My love life was an absolute mess. I can say this now to describe the young "me" back then, I had really shitty taste in men. The caliber of which wasn't surprising at all in hindsight. They had to be handsome, intelligent, wealthy, successful and older than me. All that to deserve a part of me I didn't even believe in myself. I was especially attracted to the distant, hard to get, and unavailable. I thought it was hot. I put up with so much shit because my own self-respect was in the toilet. Pun intended.

The expensive gifts, exotic vacations, jewelry, limos rides, private plane rides to another state and back again for dinner.... meh.

I received very little emotionally from them in return. That was the hook, which perpetuated the longing for more...that I was never going to have. Knock-knock, hello? Are you in there? Lol!

I couldn't seem to bond or get close with anyone long enough to have a relationship. There was always that void of intimacy between us that I didn't know how to fill. I couldn't even begin to recognize what was missing anyway. If they turned out to be sweet and nice, that was especially a big turn-off; I didn't respect that. Bye-bye! I remember feeling lonely most of the time. Welcome to my early twenties.

CHAPTER TWENTY-THREE

Dark Days

Speaking of boyfriends, here's a story about a friend of mine who had a very good-looking and sweet boyfriend. Except for one teeny little flaw not obvious early in the relationship. His name was Jimmy.

It still cracks me up every time I think about this one.

Being a doctor, I often get phone calls at home from my friends and family with health concerns and for advice. My friend, Joanna, called me late one evening worried about her right foot. It started off as a slight ache in the morning, but as the day progressed it got considerably worse. She could not recall any precipitating factors or injuries that would make her foot hurt so badly. She described the foot pain as throbbing, cold, and too painful to walk on. I thought it might be an arterial obstruction, and advised her to go to the emergency room. Joanna worked for the hospital and dreaded the thought of being in the ER. I then suggested we try EFT on it.

Knowing Joanna as well as I do, I was careful not to step on her "other foot. " That's the topic of her boyfriend, Jimmy. She had spent the weekend with him, and his quirky ways frequently frustrate her. I also knew she had some anger attached to past experiences with him, so I began tapping with her, gingerly.

"Even though I'm angry, I deeply and completely accept myself." Keeping it general the first round decreased the pain from a 10 to a 7.

The second round was more specific.

"Even though I have anger in my right foot because I can't express it and I have to put it someplace, I deeply and completely love and accept myself." That brought the pain down to a 4.

She was completely surprised that her foot felt warm and that the pain had decreased quite a bit! Joanna admitted that she'd been angry at Jimmy all day. As sweet as he is, he has a real problem with road rage. He had scared the heck out of her, almost causing an accident.

So our last round went "Bitch Tap" style (tap and tell him off) to get her power back!

"I'm pissed off at Jimmy, and it's in my damn right foot!" "I've been wanting to kick him in the fucking ass all day!" We both started to laugh out loud, but I encouraged her to continue her rant and get it all out. "You son-of-a-bitch, you could have killed us both! What the fuck is wrong with you? Get some help, bitch! I hate your ass right now!"

Of course, she was so scared and stunned during her car ride with him, she couldn't say those things in the moment. She stuffed it down, and guess where it landed? Stewing about it all day, she had the urge to give him a swift kick in the ass! And now, Joanna had gotten her nut. Sigh, another day for me at the office! Lol!

She was in shock and awe that her foot pain was completely gone, and it wasn't throbbing or cold either! It looked and felt normal again. She was so grateful that she could get some sleep for work early the next morning. I had a funny thought before we hung up the phone. I decided we should use (tongue in cheek) medical terminology for her mysterious foot pain. She had a bad case of "Jimmy Foot!"

<u>Nothing like an emotional expression of a "boot in the ass" to clear things out! LOL!</u>

They lasted a few more months after this until she finally slammed the breaks on their romance. Pun intended!

Caution; Someone with road rage (unexpressed anger) is not concerned with passenger safety. It means they don't mind taking you with them on the ride to hell when a stranger in another vehicle pisses them off. If you ride with someone you know has these issues, it's a mistake as serious as getting into a car with a drunk driver. You relinquish your control over personal safety to someone who is completely out of control. If this applies to you, the issues around this topic (self-destruction) is well worth a closer look at your self-work.

While I enjoyed free flights anywhere Continental flew, and loved living near the beach in Los Angeles, I avoided going home to Indiana. In hindsight, I was meant to be away for my own growth; in fact, that's the way mom raised me. And a cloistered family life with mommy and daddy weighing in on my every move was out of the question.

And then, the unthinkable happened to all of us. My brother, Louie, estranged from my parents, died from a drug overdose. He was only 27 years old when he left us all behind. Our entire family was devastated. We took it very hard.

Aside from his very obvious physical beauty, that shock of curly black hair, and his fine-featured face of a Spaniard, Louie was born a musical savant. He had an "ear" for music, a photographic auditory memory for sounds. With very few formal lessons, he taught himself how to play and master every instrument he ever laid his hands on. From woodwinds to strings, harps, xylophones, his drum skills were epic. He wrote music for every instrument in a symphony. He studied music composition at Indiana University, Bloomington. He was a natural born artist exactly like my mom. He excelled especially in the art of figure drawing and caricatures. From the time he was a little kid, he would keep my cousins and I endlessly entertained. We laughed at his hilarious family sketches that poked fun at aunts, uncles, and us. Nobody was safe from his naughty little poison pencil. The one great love of his life was a beautiful Irish girl who was his high school sweetheart. They were very young when they married because she was pregnant. They had a beautiful dark-haired daughter with her father's eyes that he could never, ever feel worthy of. He was ill-prepared to be a good father or ever to become a balanced, mature man. He would later cancel himself out of her life and give her up for adoption when his ex-wife remarried. It was his greatest sorrow in life.

He was quick-witted, and a teaser, sarcastic, bless his heart, and funny. He had a brilliant mind and was so gifted with artistic talents. It was his enormous amount of unfulfilled potential that shattered my heart into a million tiny little pieces when he passed away. It was a very hard and painful loss because, to me, he went to his grave feeling unloved and unsupported. At least, that's what I thought at the time. Tons of EFT years later, I was wrong about that too. His memory still resides in a special place inside my heart, just as young and beautiful and as funny as he ever was. As for the rest of our precious times together when we were kids, I'll take those with me when I go. Even though I never knew how to begin to express it to him during the time he was with us, I adored him.

I lived in California now, I was far away from home. So for five hard years, after he died, I mourned his loss silently and inwardly. I didn't tell anyone, it was too big to talk about. Louie and I never had the opportunity to talk to each other about our early experiences together. What happened to us, how we felt about it. I was too busy licking my own wounds, trying to find balance, trying to recover on my own the best way I knew how. At the same time, I was scraping together every piece of self-respect I could muster on my own, and it was a slow crawl. I couldn't even begin to take on his anger and sadness too. It took me many, many years before I could allow myself to think about the emotional toll it took on Louie. It hurt too badly to look at it honestly, so for years, I didn't look at it at all. In the end, it was intricately tied to my own healing.

I was left with a tremendous amount of guilt because he was so terribly damaged. I didn't know how to protect him, and I was angry with him because he didn't know how to defend me either. I always wanted him to be the type of big brother who was protective and defended me. But he never could, especially for himself. I forgave this entire complexed web of emotions eventually using EFT to do it. I can talk about him now without my throat tightening, it no longer hurts to talk about him at all.

CHAPTER TWENTY-FOUR

The Gift

There is a time to mourn, and it should be honored as an individual need for each person and a normal reaction. But what if its life-altering and paralyzing, keeping you stuck? Excessive feelings of any emotion wear down your immune system, eventually making you sick. Ever hear of "She died of a broken heart? This is a true story about a sad and tortured woman. She used to drive her friend to our office for Chiropractic treatments. This is how she was suddenly set free after she accepted the help of EFT, a technique she knew nothing about at the time, but was open and willing to try.

<u>I am so grateful for Debbie's willingness to accept my gift to her, which I don't usually impose. But, in this case, I was strongly compelled by my inner voice to approach her. I am so glad I listened.</u>

As I've mentioned, we had a chiropractic practice in a small town in Southwest Michigan. We had a patient who would occasionally be driven to her appointments by a friend of hers named Debbie. Debbie's appearance was one of a person who looked lost. She would sit quietly and wait for her friend with her eyes cast downward. Actually, she avoided all eye contact with anyone else in the waiting room.

Since we weren't from Michigan, unbeknown to us, Debbie had a tragic story which was, by now, common knowledge in our small town. In September of 1991, Debbie's oldest son, Anthony, was fishing in rough waters off the pier in town on Lake Michigan when he was swept away by a wave. His body was discovered a week later. He was seventeen years old.

One day Debbie actually came in to see us as a patient, looking even worse than I ever remembered. I was compelled to ask what was wrong as she sat in the waiting room looking very small and teary-eyed. She said it was the day before the anniversary of her son Anthony's death. It was always an excruciatingly painful time for her. In fact, all the holidays, including his birthday, were especially brutal. Sixteen years after his death her response to his memory was now ritualistic. This included day-long graveside vigils sitting on the ground and sobbing. I sat next to her and held her hand and asked her if she would accept a gift from me. Blinking through tears, barely able to speak, she nodded "yes."

I began with the painfully obvious and worked my way forward.

"Even though my entire being can't accept the fact that you're gone, I love and accept who I am, and I honor myself for trying to keep you with me." Reminder phrase 1st round; "I can't believe you're gone, I won't believe it." 2nd round, "I'll dishonor your memory if I let you go, I'm afraid to let go."

"I accept myself even though a part of me died with you." Reminder phrase; "A part of myself is gone forever, you didn't die alone, mom died too."

"Even though I'll never get over the way you died, I choose to be grateful for our time together and celebrate your life."

Reminder phrase: 1st round of "I'll never get over the way you died."

2nd round: "I'm so grateful you were born, and I'll celebrate your life," "I'm so happy I had you as long as I did."

With each of those phrases, Debbie released big sighs of relief and was amazed by how much better she felt, how relaxed she was. We had now unleashed a steady flow of memories, so I followed her lead. She said "I had this recurring dream every night before they found him. We're both together in the water trying to reach for each other's hands while he's calling out to me for help---and no matter how hard I try, I can't reach his hand. I still have them regularly; it takes me days to shake it off".

I usually refrain from using religious connotations during sessions, out of respect for my clients who represent a variety of different faiths. In her case, I used the language of her faith. Debbie is a deeply religious Christian.

"Even though I couldn't reach out far enough to save you, I trust you took the hand of Jesus, and he safely led you home." Reminder phrase; "I couldn't save you, but Jesus did," "You're safe in the hands of Jesus," "Handing you over to Jesus, and trusting in the Lord."

With that round, she exclaimed she felt elated. No matter how she tested it, couldn't seem to replicate the terrible guilt and sadness that she'd been feeling for years. "Actually, I feel a flood of warmth wash over me-- almost like warm water being poured over my head, and a tingling rush of energy all through my arms and legs!"

Now Debbie was crying again, but this time with relief. She said that she felt light as a feather and hugged me. And for the first time I saw a smile on her face that was so bright, it was as if the sun was bursting out from behind a dark cloud. Her eyes were gleaming as she said goodbye and bounded out of the room. Since the next day was the anniversary of her son's death, I asked her to give me a call and let me know how she was doing.

Instead, the next day she stopped by the clinic on her way home from the cemetery, and she had the most beautiful smile on her face! Her energies were completely different. She was bouncy and upbeat! Debbie happily announced that she took flowers and balloons and released them as a celebration of his life. This instead of sitting all day on a blanket at his gravesite, crying and grieving as she did for the past 16 years.

"Thank you from the bottom of my heart for your gift to me, Dr. Rossanna." This time my eyes were welling up with tears. As I tapped to regain my composure, I made her promise to periodically check back with me as the holidays were approaching.

Right before Christmas, I received a very animated phone call from Debbie. For the first time since Anthony's death, she actually decorated her own Christmas tree without being coaxed by her family. And she enjoyed it immensely! Filled with the Christmas spirit, she pulled out the old ornaments he made in school and hung them on the tree in his honor because he loved Christmas too. "This Christmas feels so wonderfully different," she said. "It's always been my favorite time of the year"! "I can't believe how good I feel! Merry Christmas to you Dr. Rossanna, God bless you".

Imagine the enormity of EFT's impact, illustrated here by such a positive and powerful emotional shift in one brief session.

After 16 years of excessive grief, it's gone in twenty minutes.

Grief, with it's varying stages, is a normal process. EFT does not erase new grief or even make you forget the subject you're grieving for. What it does do is desensitize excessive, panicky grief--the kind that makes you want to die, too. Because it is a self-help tool, we are now capable of having an easier transition to life re-adjusted. An easier, kinder, and a gentler way to reach inner peace and the clarity to move on with our lives.

Since we've moved away from Michigan, Debbie is my FaceBook friend. She periodically sends me good tidings, and pictures of the new loves in her life--her precious, grandchildren. God is good.

As for me, I know in my heart that my big brother, Louie, is at peace. Besides, he has a lot of very good company in the afterlife. My entire family is very comfortable with the feeling of "knowing" that to be true.

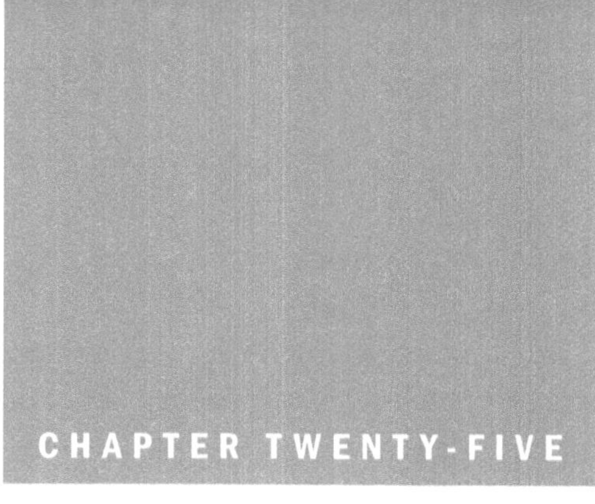

Beyond the Veil

We grew up right next door to the house my dad, and ten of his siblings were born and raised. His two infant brothers and a bed-ridden teenage sister, Evelyn, died in that house. So did both of his middle-aged parents, who passed away one year apart. And later, when my Uncle George owned the house, his wife, Barbara, died there after a long illness. Uncle George, who smoked a cigar, still lived in the family home when he passed away.

Our entire family, cousins included, have a deep connection to our Esper family home, the house next door. My own family grew accustomed to living in and around both houses. We discovered there were many spirits attached to them.

It wasn't unusual for psychic phenomenon to occur in our house, and the family house next door. It wasn't uncommon at all. We could hear knocking on interior doors, and see doorknobs turn and doors open. No one was ever there that we could see. We instinctively knew it was dad's family. There were olfactory hauntings of cigar smoke, and sometimes, the smell of roses. We even had auditory hauntings of a small dog barking in our kitchen at night. Even my dad saw "ectoplasm" forming upstairs next door where he stored his things. He asked it; "Is that you mama?" He got spooked and ran down the stairs saying his feet never touched the ground! After a while, we grew comfortable knowing our family was watching over us from the other side.

On separate occasions, my sister and I saw an apparition of a young man in our bedroom. He wore clothes from the 1890's with garters on both arms over his shirtsleeves. He made motions with his hands as if he wanted us to follow him. Okay, that was scary. Lol! Mom would have our house blessed by a priest more than once for good measure. We never saw the apparition again.

My dad was born with a veil over his face, a birth **caul.** [5] His mother saved it for him in a box as a "sign" signifying her child was born with a predominant psychic gift.

No doubt about it, dad is "psychic." He can "see" a person within minutes of being in their presence. Good or bad intentions, he knows right away, and he's never shy about expressing it, right in the moment. If we thought we had any secrets from dad, we were wrong! As adults, if need be, he forewarns us about ominous events or the people in our lives. And he's always right. And we listen.

Us cousins on dad's side of the family all have very closely woven psychic ties together. More than one of us can see our departed, hear them, or both, or in my case, they come to us in dreams.

So far, it's only been my Syrian relatives, more recently, my brother Louie, who comes to me in visitation dreams. Some of them come to explain unfinished business to set the record straight. Some come so I can tell family members they're okay, young again, and without health problems anymore. I've done that for my family for as long as I can remember. We all accept it as normal. There are times when they forewarn of someone's passing, and that helps us to prepare. My own blessing, dad's sister and our family matriarch, Aunt Margie, and her husband, Uncle Ralph, come without fail to see me in my dreams. As they did in life, they're always there to cheer me on during important personal events. The night before a project launch or other major events, one or both come to visit and encourage. That phenomenon feels very normal and natural to me. I'm so grateful for our close connection. True love between us never dies, and our Syrian family remains strongly connected, and very close.

Back to my journey and how I made my way back to dad. Now that my brother was gone, I found my dad even less tolerable to be around.

---

[5] (Latin name, Caput galeatum, meaning "head helmet"), is a piece of the amniotic sac still attached to a newly **born baby's** head or face. https://en.wikipedia.org/wiki/Caul

I would wait for him to step out of line so I could crush him with my anger. It got so bad that after a rare visit, I realized that all my rage was lost on him. I also realized that screaming at him not only made him feel bad, it also made me feel worse. It didn't feel good to hurt him, it felt horrible. It wasn't rational communication anyway, it was irrational. Acting like him did nothing to improve our communication skills together. We were stuck in the past leaning into negative familiar behavioral patterns. I was vibrating rage, and doing my best imitation of dad. Disgusted with myself, I called him from the airport on my way back home to California. I apologized to him. I was so sorry I hurt him. I diminished him in the moment, and it didn't feel satisfying, it just plain sucked. I confess it ended up being a bitter victory. It's a horrible feeling to over-power someone like that. That was never the real me inside, yet I delivered my worst reaction. I don't intentionally hurt people, ever. My aggressive reaction and bad behavior heightened my anxiety levels. It took me weeks to shake off my visit home.

CHAPTER TWENTY-SIX

Shake It Off

With every interaction, we exchange traces of energy. Be it animal or human, we can feel it in a positive, or a negative way. For our own health, it's not our energy to keep unless, of course, it's positive and uplifting. Who needs the stress of extra baggage?

For healthcare practitioners and "people helpers," the wide range of "people drama" throughout the course of a day leaves an imprint. It also applies to anyone who feels affected being around negative, saturating energies. This could be difficult family members or persnickety friends we put up with but love just the same. Whatever the case may be, EFT is a powerful way to deflect and lower your stress levels with people interactions every day.

Early on in my EFT practice, I noticed that I couldn't stop thinking about my client's issues after a session. I needed to make a conscious effort to shake off my client's energies since I take it on and still see it. Seeking advice from some of the EFT Masters at a workshop, they told me several ways to center myself before a session. That didn't work. It finally dawned on me to try EFT in-between client sessions. After all, Gary said: "try it on everything." And it worked great. Which leads to my excitement in sharing this wisdom.

Because my EFT specialty is serious diseases, I'm exposed to the energies of people with huge psychological reversals. My clients almost always ask me how I handle the potential energy drain of so many issues. They are always surprised to hear that I use EFT on myself after our sessions. This also helps reinforce the power and healing potential of EFT in the minds of my clients. Because of the complexity and seriousness of the diseases I deal with, my sessions usually last an hour. More than enough time to be bombarded with negativity. With a quick round or two of EFT after each session, I'm clear and focused on my next client. In the long run, it helps ensure the clarity and quality of my work.

Here are some prime examples of my basic set-up and reminder phrases I routinely use after each session. I always test between rounds, and if need be, repeat until I can no longer piece the individual "scenes" together to make any sense.

Since everyone releases energy differently, I urge you to rely on your own testing techniques for best results. It's good to start with the general tone of each client session--anger, grief-filled, traumatic, depressive, and so on.

"I accept myself even though I've picked up Jane Doe's depressed/sad/angry energy;" RP (reminder phrase): "Releasing Jane's depressed energies."

*Tip: Go back through your session with Jane Doe. Replay the movie, grab whatever part of the memory of their issue you still have, and tap until it's released.

Set up phrases for family and friends will follow the same course. Here are more examples. Remember to do this the same day of energetic exposure for immediate results.

"Even though I'm affected by my dad/mom's depressed energies, I deeply love and accept myself."

RP: "Releasing dad/mom's depressed energy."

"I take it personally; it's about his/her own issues and not mine."

"Even though my sister/brother's anger permeates the room and effects me negatively, I deeply love and accept myself."

"Releasing sister/brother's anger energies."

"Even though my friend constantly complains and brings me down when I'm with her, I remember the things I love about her."

RP: "Shaking off Rosemary's residue."

The best thing about shaking off other people's energies is that it is entirely possible to enjoy a healthy emotional balance on a daily basis. Imagine how much better an ER doctor or nurse might feel at the end of the day using EFT to emotionally shake off the experiences of each work shift? Perhaps the label: the "wounded healer," would become an old and irrelevant phrase. The possibilities are excitingly endless.

Candace Pert [6]has suggested that we're all hard-wired for bliss. The very young, before the "writing on their walls" [7] get too filled with clutter, seem to express their state of "bliss" much of the time. Perhaps this means that our own personal state of daily bliss is not quite as elusive as we may think. Use EFT throughout the day, when and as the effects of "life and others" disturb our energies. This allows for the possibility of achieving a healthful state of inner balance. Something all of us are "hardwired" for.

<u>This is my EFT after-exposure ritual, and an essential tool for a happy, balanced, daily life.</u>

---

[6] Molecules of Emotion, https://www.amazon.com/Molecules-Emotion-Science-Mind-Body-Medicine/dp/0684846349

[7] A metaphor commonly used by Gary Craig to reference all the learnings, programming, beliefs, etc. that our minds accumulate as we grow into adults

CHAPTER TWENTY-SEVEN

Once Upon a Chiropractor

After ten years of flying, living in Houston, Denver, and Los Angeles, and ending in long commutes from Oakland, California to Houston, I had enough. The airline industry drastically changed, the passengers changed, and it just felt like drudgery. I felt worn out and unfulfilled. Although I loved the people I worked with and quitting meant not working with my cousin anymore, I just couldn't stay, I wasn't feeling it. I took an early out option with lifetime flight benefits and hung up my wings in 1985.

I longed to finish what I started back at Indiana University, and go back to school. Mama always said a pretty face is a dime a dozen, but a female with a professional degree and a career is a full-on game-changer. In a completely different direction than my last more "glamorous" profession, I wanted to become a doctor. Not just any doctor mind you. I had an extraordinary "one minute wonder" manual (by hand) adjustment from a Chiropractor when I was seven years old. That experience was as much a part of my career decision as the exposure to our family home remedies from my grandmother and my mom. It laid the groundwork for my interest in the ancient natural healing arts. The message being, as in nature, given the proper support, the body can heal itself.

Back to my Chiropractic drama story. Mom had a tree surgeon hang a long, thick, knotted rope for us kids to swing on from one of our old, giant, cottonwood trees in the backyard. We leaned a ladder up against the tree and take turns leaping onto the rope. Like Tarzan, me Jane, as the rope swung back to the ladder, the next person waiting had to jump off the ladder and catch it. We were like trapeze artists catching the rope, while other people were still hanging on. The goal was to see how many of us could swing on the rope at the same time.

One summer evening, like fleas in a circus with our Fulton Street cousins, we were swinging on the rope. Brother Louie, always the jokester, decided to increase the challenge further by making us laugh. Ad-libbing funny lyrics to a popular song, and making funny noises, as much as we tried not to, we all started laughing hysterically. My hands were the first to slip off the rope, and I dropped from mid-air to the ground landing flat on my stomach. Everyone fell off too, some of them landing directly on top of my back. Ouch.

I had the wind knocked out of me and was panic-stricken because as much as I tried, I couldn't breathe. Gasping for breath and crawling on my hands and knees, I tried my best to make it back to the house for help.

I'll never forget what happened during my death crawl. I actually saw my entire life flash before my eyes. Okay, I was only 7 years old when it happened, so it wasn't a very long flash. But it was to the minute detail. Every single individual life event moved like a fast, but easy to see motion picture reel in my mind's eye. I even remember seeing the animal print of the nursery curtains. That was weird to me because I had by then, forgotten all about them until I saw them again. It was a very strange and wondrous experience that did not feel scary at all. I'd have another near-death experience again many years later in a whitewater rafting accident...but that's another story.

Back to my drama story, mom ran out of the house, helped me to my feet, and walked me around until I finally caught my breath. We had company over, so after seeing everyone so alarmed, I played it off. I was just fine, I told them, and I refused an emergency room visit. I was terrified of white coats, medical doctors, shots, needles, more pain, and the smell of a medical facility, eww, the alcohol smell. I was successful at faking it, and I won that round. Whew!

The downside to that was I suffered in silence for weeks because my low back was absolutely killing me. When it became visibly evident I was in pain, and I couldn't hide it anymore, I was in for more fear.

Everyone started telling mom that I probably had kidney damage. I'd probably have to go to the hospital, and I'd probably have to have surgery. It was absolutely terrifying for me to hear. I begged her not to take me to the hospital.

I can thank my lucky stars that my mom was no ordinary mom. She was a gifted musician who taught herself to play piano by ear when she was a little girl, and she was also an artist and prolific writer. Self-educated with many interests, mom's biggest passion was holistic healing and nutrition. Using her mother's remedies, she healed our childhood illnesses. She would rub our head bumps back down with butter and a flat butter knife, or make us drink mint tea or eat barley soup for tummy aches. Lung issues were treated with hot enchiladas to make you sweat (capsicum induced capillary dilatation) and break a head cold. Her own mother came from twelve generations (four centuries) of female healers. They're known in Latin communities as Curanderas. Grandmother's family fled Ledesma, a small Medieval village in the Salamanca province of Castile and Leon, Spain. They ended up settling in Acapulco, Mexico, bringing with them midwifery and ancient bone setting techniques. They also made potions and practiced spiritual cures handed down to them in Spain by the Greeks, Romans, and Moors.

My grandmother used indigenous plants, roots, food, teas, and other remedies to heal. That came in handy to stitch together the childhood wounds of her 10 children. People in the neighborhood and family friends came to her. She set broken bones, reduced dislocations, massaged and manipulate the spine by hand. They also came for wound healing and midwifery. She knew how to manually turn a breech baby into the proper position for an easier birth. She made her own salves and ointments from indigenous Southwestern herbs. She knew how to heal wounds, grow hair, sooth muscles, and calm nerves. Astute in her wisdom, grandmother was well versed. That type of collection from ancient wisdom is called Curanderia Entero. That basically means, she didn't specialize in just one way to heal someone, she did it all.

Choosing what was best for me ultimately, thank God, mom went with her gut instincts. She bypassed the threatening medical doctor visit with our family doctor, Boris Karloff. Instead, she took me to see a good old-fashioned bone mover, and friendly neighborhood Chiropractor, Dr.

Wooten. My first office visit happened quickly. I had to see for myself he had nothing in his hands that could hurt me like a 20-foot long needle attached to a big ugly glass syringe. Dr. Wooten was a big man. In a low, calm, voice he asked me to lay on my back. As he bent my top leg over my bottom leg to put me into a side posture, told me to inhale deeply, and before I could finish exhaling all the way, boom! I heard the audible sounds of my joints release, or "cracking" as laypeople call it, actually a gas release within the joints. I felt instant relief and was suddenly pain-free after weeks of excruciating pain. After intense suffering in silence, my back felt warm and tingly. It was my Chiropractic miracle and my doctor's one-minute wonder. I got up from the table and asked, is that all? And we all had a bit of a chuckle. It was exactly what I needed. Thank you doc, bravo, nice work! Years later I would learn that children respond and heal to Chiropractic adjustments much more quickly than adults. Imagine that?

The Trouble With Angels

I returned to college and finished my prerequisites. I chose to attend Life Chiropractic College-West, in San Lorenzo, California. Chiropractic college was both exhilarating and challenging. I made life-long friendships with many of my wonderful classmates. And it's where I met my best friend, bookend, cohort, and fellow fashionista/doctor, Wendi Marks.

Wendi's father, Norman Marks, also a Chiropractor, was a part of "The Physical Culture" (aka bodybuilding trend) of the 1940's. Inspired by his longtime friend, mentor, and fitness legend, Jack LaLanne, Norman won Mr. America in 1946 and in 1947. He then won Mr. California in 1948. Owner of "Norman Marks Health Club," Wendi was going to practice Chiropractic with him at the health club after she graduated.

It was my first up-close and personal look at a different kind of father-daughter relationship. You could just see the love he had for Wendi, and her sister, Rhonda. He was fiercely proud of them, I loved seeing the look in his eyes when he spoke to them, they said it all. The funny thing is, it didn't make me feel sad or jealous, it was great to be around to see that type of father-daughter love was really possible, I was happy for them.

In jest she would later say it was to keep her enemies closer, Wendi and I became fast friends the moment we met each other in class. Two peas in a pod, let's just say we weren't the typical Birkenstock wearing, patchouli smelling, bare-faced earth mothers in school. We were all about the late 80's current fashion trends, big hair, shoulder pads, mini skirts, high heels and statement earrings. Not exactly schoolgirl uniforms, our clothes were a different feminist testimony. Femininity and professionalism come in all shapes and sizes. Our message was there's no shame in being smart and looking pretty. We were just being ourselves, which meant clomping down the halls in 2-3 inch heels for a typical day at school was our normal. Oye! I got over it, I very rarely wear those bio-mechanically incorrect instruments of torture now.

Wendi and I had a friendly academic competition between us. It kept us focused and pushed our capacity for learning the new language of the human body. And learn we did, memorizing the names of every bone, tissue, organ, nerve enervation, muscular origins and insertions. We learned how to read x-rays and how to recognize pathologies, and so much more.

Our Zen moments together between classes were shopping at our favorite hangout, Macy's Warehouse. It was our regular reward for a long day, and a way to decompress after a big exam. I'll never forget our times together, she was always so funny and mischievous, our favorite thing to do was laugh. In turn, she would say I was her evil twin, but hey, my book, my way! As naughty school girls together, she played Mary Clancy to my Rachel like in the 1966 movie, "The Trouble With Angels." I was the innocent one I'm telling ya! Lol! We're still very close soul sisters to this day.

Life-West offered free psychological counseling, by counseling psychology interns, for any students in need. Life-West was a progressive and student sensitive college. It was a wonderful service for those of us who lacked coping skills. I took an accelerated curriculum option to shave off an entire year of school by going year round with little or no breaks from class time in between. The stress from taking 13 classes per quarter was at first very intense for me. It started to trigger repressed memories that seemed to pop up out of nowhere.

It became so distracting that I decided to take that first step and seek counseling. After interviewing several interns, I chose a female therapist. She was a published author who wrote a book about astral projection of all things. That got my attention because as a small child during nap time, I would regularly practice levitating out of my body. To get in "the zone" I would focus on the ceiling and touch it with my nose. I could count the decorative holes in the ceiling tile, and float around the room. I could softly leap down our staircase and back again without ever feeling the weight of gravity or touching the steps. I could repeat that process, every single nap time and looked forward to doing it! Thinking it was normal, I never told anyone, but I certainly enjoyed it while it lasted. Before I met my therapist, I never knew there was a name for it. She was open-minded, kind, caring, comfortable to be around, and non-threatening, I trusted her. It would be the first time I ever shared the really bad secrets, including the "babysitter" and the first time I ever voiced them out loud to anyone, ever.

The cognitive behavioral therapy offered intellectual catharsis and emotional validation. It helped me to be more sensitive to my own inner feelings and for once, entitled to have them. It was there that I learned how to cry again, which was at first so humiliating. I hated for her to see me cry those first bitter tears. It meant weakness, a chink in the armor, and it was a tough, hard rule for me to break. But crying was a huge victory in my treatment. I saw her for several months until we felt the stress issues had resolved. I certainly felt much calmer, more balanced, and I got through the rest of school without a hitch.

The California Chiropractic State Board exams, the toughest in the nation, didn't scare me a bit. I passed all three days of written, practical and oral exams. Turns out, dad was wrong; I wasn't so stupid after all. Duh!

Love Wins

Meanwhile, back to my EFT experiment, you know, the one where I was applying it to myself to see if this stuff really worked? It was that second going-over using EFT on my oldest and worst childhood memories that finished collapsing the residual junk.

This time, I targeted the same issues I worked on with Cognitive Behavioral Therapy, back as a student. The deep shame, the hatred, the anger, and sadness; all the stuff I thought I had let go of before, was now resolved at a deep, cellular level. And for the sake of inner personal peace, that's where it counts.

I forgave my dad for hurting us, for hurting me, with all my heart, and I really, truly, meant it with all my heart. Easier still, I forgave myself too with all my heart for hurting him all those years after the fact, and for the shame of feeling justified in doing it. The war was over. I never fought with or disrespected my dad ever again, and our relationship healed completely. The best thing about it for me was that for the first time in our lives together, we were finally able to relax and enjoy each other's company. Now we could laugh together, something we both have in common and love to do.

Several years later, I helped my dad write a letter to the Veterans Administration to apply for 100% disability. That's when I learned the real truth about what dad went through in the service. He was a 24-year-old sailor with a head injury, floating out in the middle of nowhere on a destroyer in the South Pacific, a bazillion miles away from home.

A few years after his medical discharge, he met and married my mom. He kept his physical problems to himself (that's why no hearing aids) because he thought there were other soldiers worse off than he was. He received 20% disability already, so he soldiered on, and kept his mouth shut about his problems. Remember I said the only thing I knew about dad was that he was in the Navy, a little hard of hearing, and he wore this thing in his mouth called a partial? This is what his reality looked like back then, unbeknown to us. He suffered daily headaches, blurred vision, and bouts of double vision. The worst, in his opinion, was the constant, pounding pain in his ears. He heard shrill, whistling noise like a gust of wind that blew relentlessly inside his head 24 hours a day. Even worse than that, it wouldn't go away while he was asleep. At best, he could only get about three hours of sleep a night, a pattern of insomnia he had the rest of his adult life, and a source of lifelong agitation. He struggled with chronic depression and daily anxiety. Until he admitted it, none of us knew he fought back thoughts of suicide.

My dad really did soldier on. He owned his own barber shop, cut hair; his "crew cuts" and "flat tops" were legendary. He went to work every day of his life to support us no matter what. With the unknown amount of physical discomfort he had on a daily basis, I don't recall him ever taking a sick day to stay home, never, ever. Thanks to dad, as he would say, we all ate "like kings" at home, we never had to worry about not having enough of anything. When I look back at it now, it's incredible how he'd find the time and the money to maintain everything to take a month off of work for our family vacation. Every single summer he would drive mom and us four kids to El Paso so she could be together with her parents and the rest of her family. Our road-food on those long car trips, thanks to mom, were epic culinary adventures to remember. We always started off with Syrian food.

As a barber during the 60's and 70's when long hair was the thing, haircuts were fewer and far between. But my dad hung in there and showed up for work the whole time, undaunted; he kept on 'truckin'. We knew all his regular customers loved him. One friend, Jerry Davis, (the egg man) brought lunch and eggs to him once a week for many years just so they could eat together and visit at the shop. His barbershop was the town meeting place for men. Along with their haircuts, they came to exchange business advice and to seek wise counsel from dad. If they were lucky, they also could get two cents worth of advice from the variety of professional men who were his regular customers. It's so nice to know my dad was so appreciated and well respected as the best barber in town.

There wasn't a name for what was going on with dad back when my brother Louie and I were living at home. As small children, our primitive little hindbrains (amygdala) called it "dad doesn't love me, dad hates my guts." He didn't fit the stereotypical "shell-shocked" soldier affect of the old 1940's war movies. None of us had any idea, we just thought dad was mean. Hit by a shell casing that slammed into his brain, dad had a very long recovery. The aftermath of a closed head injury (severe concussion) is brain swelling. Because of the damage to his right inner ear that left him deaf, dad rebounded by becoming expert at lip reading. It wasn't until he received his 100% disability that he finally got fitted for hearing aids. Include in the mix his traumatic hospitalization experience for six months. All together it added up to something we never knew existed.

There's a name for it now, it's called PTBIS (Post Traumatic Brain Injury Syndrome.)

For the record, both PTBIS and PTSD (Post Traumatic Stress Disorder) are easily handled by a very special feature in EFT.

It uses therapeutic dissociation, a method called "The Tearless Trauma Technique." It happens without ever having to talk about it or go through it again. It's completely pain-free (tearless), fast-acting and drama free. Have I mentioned this stuff works?

I'm so grateful that (even though he didn't know what to make of it) dad was gracious enough to tap with me. We worked through all memories he could think of starting with the story of his head injury. We got through the difficult treatments he endured during his hospitalization too. An avid and excellent bowler and golfer, I taught him how to tap for performance empowerment. He used it as his secret weapon to beat his golf and bowling buddies time and time again! He told me how he would tap while inside his truck beforehand so nobody would see him and think he was acting crazy! Lol, that's my paw!

For the record, I have two younger siblings who did not share the same traumatic experiences we had. They weren't born yet, and later, too young to remember. Plus dad got better with time. They went on to have entirely different relationships with both of my parents.

For the past few years now, my dad has been struggling with dementia and turns 91 this year. Mom, in perfect health, is an indomitable 87 years old. I am very grateful and very fortunate that I was able to recover and reconcile my relationship with dad.

Thank God it happened before it was too late for him to remember the fun "us" together. I'll never forget the first time I had the nerve enough to tell him I loved him after a phone conversation. In return, without missing a beat, he replied; "I love you too babe." Those words flowed easily ever after.

To make up for lost time, rather than telling them in person, I wrote my parents a personal thank you letter. I thanked them both for their contribution to my growth. Itemizing all the positive things they each taught me, I reminisced about our happy memories. I ended it by letting them each know how much I love them. I chose letter form so they could always have the words in front of them. I highly recommend personal peace, conciliation, reconciliation, and above all, forgiveness. It makes for a happy heart because it means love wins.

CHAPTER THIRTY

Swimming Upstream

Meanwhile, back at the hacienda, shortly after our move from Michigan, I received the bad news that Gary Craig was retiring. He handed over his phenomenally high profile website, Emofree.com, to Dawson Church. I felt like the rug was pulled right out from under me. Everything changed as all things do. My internet exposure, and consequently, my entire internet EFT business fell flat. It took me several months to find my bearing. I was adrift on a lifeboat at sea, without oars, and no backup plan. It was a temporary shock more than anything else, I needed time to think. I got kicked out of Gary's very comfortable referral nest, and I had to learn how to fly on my own. I admit I was spoiled! I had nothing left to do but put on my big girl chonies (pants..kind of) and reinvent. That's the good thing about sudden change, it forces you to access and ignite your own creativity.

I never gave up on how many millions of people already knew about EFT and how many of those people knew about me. I still had my global presence. It was just a matter of how to reach them now?

I decided to go in a new direction with my services and created my new website, EFTOne.com, subtitled "One Memory at a Time," because that's how you approach each specific life event. I offered free, live EFT sessions online. I created the service for people who were already experienced in tapping, but who were stuck and could use some help from a professional. It would also be an opportunity for others to see how well it works first hand. It was interesting because the only people who were game to do this online were past clients. I'm so grateful for my courageous tribe who stood by me and represented.

To protect their anonymity, we created the online meeting so that you couldn't see the client, only hear their voices. Further, I had them use a different name to help blur public recognition. In retrospect, it may have all been a little too scary for those who weren't my clients listening in. Nevertheless, it was a great experience, and it got me out of the rock I was hiding under. I knew it was the start of something bigger, but I wasn't sure exactly what that was yet.

I was also seeing private clients locally, and with George, hosting EFT Level 1 & 2 workshops. We were using a popular workshop template and slideshow written by a master EFT practitioner. We taught hundreds of people the basics and gave them the opportunity for practical experience. Along with that I also had three prime-time television interviews in El Paso under my belt. We assumed from our workshops that they easily picked up the technique and used it. But, in follow-up conversations with my past attendees, they confessed that they weren't using it as much as I hoped they would, and some, not at all. Flustered, I called my flunky flock of past workshop attendees, my "EFT Dropouts!" I was disappointed with our track record because we apparently had blank spaces in our workshop presentation.

Whenever I had the opportunity in private, I'd ask past students to show me how they've been approaching their issues. It was always surprising to hear one of several things, and I would hear them consistently, I'll start with the top two. 1) They either were too global, and not specific enough, or 2) they stopped working on themselves because they were afraid to say the wrong thing. They weren't saying it perfectly like they thought I did. The perfection thing is a big common problem, and a core issue to work through to turn off its origin.

Getting to core events, or the origin of negative personal challenges that aren't working for you is a major tenant in EFT. Being "PERFECT" is a very common problem. Competing with God for perfection, first of all, means it's impossible. You're exhausting yourself physically from the stress of it, whether or not you're consciously aware of it. And one more thing, you don't realize how exhausting it is to be perfect all the time until you give yourself permission to give it a rest. Life gets 1000 times lighter!

Defusing the emotional driver of "perfection" is a topic of a Storyboard list all its own. It requires listing specific supporting events of negative experiences around not being perfect. And if you can't find supporting evidence, it could be inherited familial beliefs. Example, "If you can't do it right don't do it at all" is an excruciating tenant learned from either a perfectionist parent or a past figure of authority.

Until you buckle down and get to the core issues, you can always use generic tapping phrases that will help temporally. It will allow you to tap on other stuff without worrying you're going to mess it up and do it "wrong." Until you eventually get it right!

Choose a phrase that resonates best, like "I'm afraid to do this wrong" or "I have to do this perfect." Tap while repeating the phrase until your fear intensity has comfortably decreased. Once you feel confident enough, begin your work. But do yourself a huge favor and definitely include the perfection problem on your to-do EFT work list.

Another common mistake was saying positive setup phrases and positive reminder phrases. Nope, that's how you "want" to feel, not what you're actually feeling. I do understand how people feel safer saying positive things while tapping. But I see affirmations as an emotional force-feed. Like sucking on a piece of candy, its sweet while it lasts, but it doesn't last long. For lasting results, you have to deal with the negative emotional driver for affirmations. [8] On the other hand, favorite positive affirmations are a great way to do your own detective work to see where you're lacking. For my private clients, if they have ones that they use, I love to invert them. I turn it into a negative statement and use the negative language of EFT to find the core issues that drive the need for them. Once you deal with that, you're there!

Another complaint I heard was that it didn't work for them because the problem came back. That's usually because they didn't get the emotional intensity down to a zero thinking a low intensity was enough to turn off an issue for good...nope. It's still there, the goal is ZERO.

---

[8] There is always a negative underlying need that goes unspoken in the positive affirmation. Example: I am afraid; my affirmation would be something like: I am always brave, I am fearless.

They also didn't remember to test their results, how do you know it's gone if you don't check to see for yourself? I ask my clients when we think we're finished with an issue. I have them put their hands over their hearts, close their eyes, (center and focus) and make a positive resolution statement about their issue. It either bounces right off, or it lands with them completely. Example, "I did the best I could" or "I was a good daughter" if it's still a no, it hits immediately, and we dig back in and clean it up completely.

Lastly, they didn't consider the different "aspects" of each memory. There is always more than one emotion involved in a specific event, they shift through each event like shuffling cards. Example, you may have started off mad at someone, but now you're sad about it. And then you're mad at yourself for taking it, and then you feel guilty for your reaction and on and on. These are the aspects to look for with every event. It's important to work through each and every emotion until the entire issue is resolved.

After all my efforts, I decided that I needed to rethink the way I taught people how to approach EFT. And do it in a way that felt more natural to them without reinventing the wheel. I thought about how people usually tell their problems to friends, family and loved ones. This led me to create a couple of easier ways to used EFT without all the big formulaic combination of words to worry about getting right.

We decided to do a series of videos talking about the "EFT Dropout Syndrome." We launched an email campaign to let everyone know that I'm here to help. I want them to get the success they deserve without all the fear around the "formula," and perfection worries.

My videos were not only meant to encourage my past workshop attendees to give it another shot, but they were also geared toward another group. All the folks whose heads were spinning on overwhelm from the "Tapping Summit" on the internet.

I've talked to quite a number of people over the years who fully planned to use all the good information offered on these summits. But even though they were excited by the possibilities, it's just too much information. They never get around to actually implementing any of it. So far, that's been the standard reply.

Having said that, I think Nick Ortner has done an amazing job at marketing and getting the word out about the benefits of tapping and its uses. Thanks to him, tapping is well on the way to becoming mainstream knowledge. He's introduced it to high profile people who spread the word even further. Thanks, Nick, we needed that! Nice work! Muchas gracias!

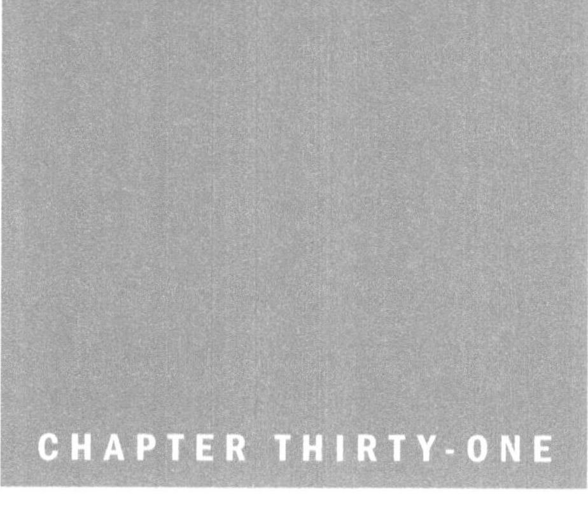

Easier Said And Done

By now, the people in my life all know me well enough to know I'm not going to sit there and listen to their personal problems for more than one time. I'm in the self-help business because I love to help people, hello? But if I listen to their negative stuff long enough, their burden becomes mine energetically. I always suggest we tap while they talk to me, and make our time together productive. At least they know they have options, and my boundaries are clear.

Who really enjoys keeping enmeshed in drama unless you're addicted to it for some reason? I see it as self-care, so I'm not afraid to admit to you that I've edited (with love) certain people out of my life who were repeat offending energy vampires. Although I do feel so much compassion for them because, in reality, they're stuck. To me, the saddest thing of all is that they can't see that they need help. It's really okay to let go of relationships that cause stress, I trust in a higher power to help them find their way out of it on their own.

Suffice it to say I do understand that misery does love company, just not with me! Not when I know life can be so beautiful without it! George and I deal with many types of personalities and a whole array of different energies at our clinic, and it's not always good energy. We maintain our personal lives and our home as drama-free zones.

The range of my experiences goes from chronic low back pain all the way to stage 4 pancreatic cancer. As you can imagine, those sessions were mostly working against the clock for a variety of reasons. You've got 6 months to live, to lab results hanging in the balance, or something vital and life-altering was about to be cut out in an upcoming surgery. For that reason, I learned how to not pussyfoot around, and to get to the core issues as quickly as possible.

For some people, the transition from thinking everything has to be verbally sorted stems from years of conditioning. Cognitive behavioral therapy was the gold standard approach to dealing with issues by talking problems out. For something new like EFT, it took years of practice talking clients down from wanting to tell me the minutia of their every problem. I got good at cutting to the chase and intuiting where to go first. I devised shortcuts, secretly testing to see how little of the EFT process I could get away with. And you want to know something? I got away with a lot. I developed two different approaches to the solution. The first is called "Grumble Tap."

This approach evolved out of my experiences with several family members who simply could not get the concepts of EFT and insisted on telling me (as if talk therapy) every gory detail of the past memory. Finally, out of frustration I forcefully told them to at least TAP while telling me the endless details. To say the least, EFT worked! They would sigh, yawn, shiver, belch...all the indicators of a physical release response. So, it's as simple as talking while tapping...get it? Instead of trying to remember the classic formula, and all the fear around not saying it right, just talk, and tap.

For extra measure, to make sure you focus on the issue, you could also start the tapping round by saying; "I'll never forget the time when..." and fill in your story. Of course, you should test your results between each round of tapping. Record the remaining intensity level, if for nothing else, so you can see with your own eyes that the intensity is, in fact, going down. And you're doing it yourself! Repeat until the intensity is at a zero. It's that simple.

It turns out, self-love and acceptance are entirely different issues. So I often omit the traditional EFT self-acceptance statement altogether. I've found that it's deserving its own Storyboard list for a direct route to get back to yourself. I get into more of that, in my video on self-acceptance. [9]

---

[9] You can see that video at https://EFTOne.com by registering as a member.

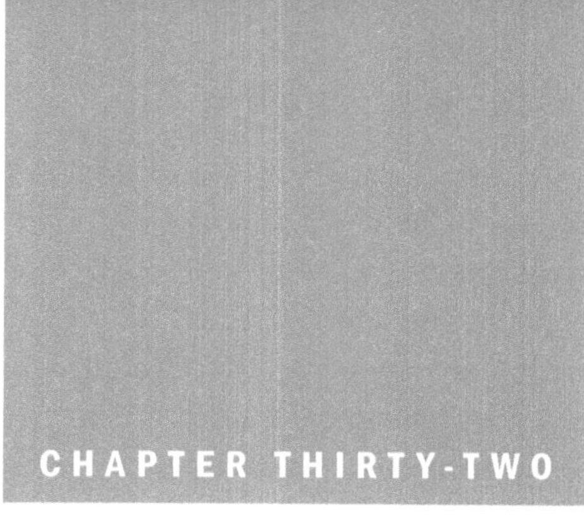

Bitch Tap Method
(Unleashing the Kraken)

I t's good manners to be sensitive about how much you unload on other people. Because, in essence, you're taking the "listener" down with the ship energetically. This leads me to my next "modification" of EFT. It's a play on the NLP (Neuro-Linguistic Programming) "power-back" technique inside EFT. I call it "Bitch Tap," a method I developed from its precursor, "The Massey Emotional Trigger Point Technique."

My beloved, late mother-in-law, Georgesther Burnett, enjoyed hearing a bit of good drama. She used to tell me; "Honey, If you don't have anything nice to say about someone, tell me everything!" I adored her, drama was entertaining for her, distracting even, but there are those of us who dread hearing it. Someone who keeps bitching about the same old issues over and over again is stuck in the past.

Bitch Tap is a personal favorite of mine, and damn fun to do, and my private clients especially love it. However, there are some people who, as they say, couldn't say shit if they had a mouthful! Cussing is encouraged in this technique which means it's going to take practice due to a blockage in the Throat Chakra. That's when I jump in and help them speak their truths when they get stuck and don't know what to say.

The breakthroughs using Bitch Tap are always extremely gratifying, surprising, and especially satisfying. It's perfect for those missed moments in life...the ones you play over and over as you beat yourself up; coulda, woulda, shoulda. You finally get your nut.

When you think about it, who couldn't use a good bitch tap? After all, life does have its ups and downs doesn't it?

This quick, crude and power-packed technique is specific for people who feel powerless. Some people have a hard time speaking up for a quick comeback in an appropriate moment. Recognize yourself yet?

What I'm calling Bitch Tap, evolved from over a decade of my experience with seriously ill clients. All who had unexpressed anger without recognizing it, and even if they did, there wasn't an effective outlet for it until this method.

And the accumulation of unexpressed anger (aka stress) sets the stage for a weakened immune system. Left unresolved, it ignites physical disease and perpetuates chronic pain syndromes.

In a nutshell, using my Bitch Tap Method™, you get your second chance at your missed moment. It works by tapping while you're bitching at the bothersome person or situation in your past, saying all the stuff you wish you did and didn't. The best thing is that if you say it in the most colorful way possible it completely gets the job done for once and for all. You finally have your say! And cussing is definitely encouraged, so "let er rip!" Speak up!

In my opinion, this is absolutely the very best way to get your power back from those missed moments in life. Those when you coulda, shoulda, woulda said something if you weren't caught off guard. There are many reasons for being stunned, afraid, or unable to speak or stand up for yourself in the moment. Many researchers believe that cussing helps to relieve stress. It actually blows off steam, just like crying does for small children. Research led by psychologist Dr. Richard Stephens [10]<u>shows</u> that cussing can actually reduce pain and make you

---

[10] http://www.mzellner.com/page4/files/2009-stephens.pdf

feel better. That's because it's closely linked to an emotionally aroused state and intense feelings.

Studies suggest that the brain processes cussing in the same regions as emotion and instinct. Bottom line, you can think of cussing as a motor activity with an emotional component. That's why you can remember cuss words about four times better than other words. Think about it, ever wonder why the first words people tend to learn and remember when learning a new language, are cuss words?

As powerful as EFT is alone, by adding cuss words while you're griping (bitching) about a bothersome issue, it helps to amp up unrecognized anger. It also provides a sharper, more intense focus resulting in an incredibly profound release! You may start off with "you're not a very nice person," but then graduate to: "you son of a bitch!" There's a huge difference when you can allow yourself to get real with your own words, and rework that missed moment this time, your way! The end result, you totally get your power back, and that's a priceless boost to your self-esteem!

On my website, I have a series of videos with live clients demonstrating how to use my Bitch Tap Method™ and as they learn how to do it you will get the right idea.

You'll see there's a great deal of tension in their throats, their "voice." That tension is what I refer to as a symptom of a Throat chakra blockage, a throat energy center, using the traditional language of Energy Medicine.

When you listen to the videos you can hear the throat tension in the way they speak, you can see the words are hard for them to come by. At that point, I'll jump in (okay, I'm good at it) and instigate a more appropriate response just to get the ball rolling.

You'll also notice not everyone is tapping in perfect sequence. That comes with a bit of experience, once you learn the tapping sequence. When you do it long enough, I encourage you to trust yourself and intuit where to tap, go where you naturally want to go. It still works as long as you're tapping on the meridian acupoints. You'll get so good at it, you'll know where it feels right for you to tap next. You might even discover a favorite place to tap, it's your special tapping G spot.

The fabulous thing about my Bitch Tap Method™ is that there is no need for a setup phrase, no reminder phrase, and no worries about doing it right or wrong. All you have to do is start bitching, and almost everyone knows how to do that, some better than others. Once you get on a roll, give that person a damn good "reading" saying every single thing you always wanted to say, and keep bitching and tapping until that #%$*!*! memory collapses completely.

Especially in the case of serious diseases and pain syndromes, people say and think horrible things about themselves. And it's that type of negative internal self-dialog that becomes so destructive to our physical bodies. In this case, I always ask my private clients if they would speak to, or treat their best friends, in the same manner they speak to and treat themselves? The answer is always "No." That's a powerful question to ask and one that always begins to reframe negative self-dialogs. My question to you is, why punish yourself and self-implode when all you have to do is bitch about the problem and tap a few acupoints?

I highly suggest you start with "you" being the focus of your anger... and bitch yourself out! Think about all those situations and all the things you've put yourself through in the past that really piss you off now. Those specific memories that keep you displeased and disappointed with yourself. Wait until you try it, you're going to feel 1000 times better! Pretty soon, you'll discover you're not so bad after all! You'll move closer in the direction to that magnificent healing power of self-love, and self-acceptance.

If you find you're having a hard time speaking your truth, baby step it at first. Just complain or grumble in your own comfortable way while you're tapping. Even if you start off whispering, at least you're forming the words internally, letting them rise up and pass through your throat and past your lips! My advice is to find a way to say what you need to say and keep moving. With diligence, you'll find yourself getting stronger and better at it, more entitled to your feelings.

Once you feel less inhibited and strong enough to flat-out bitch, in the privacy of your own home, then go ahead, throw in some F-bombs while you're at it! It'll be much, much easier and faster to hit all those negative specific events clean out of the ballpark! It's pretty cool how efficient this method is. Now you can actually bitch productively, with a positive goal in mind. The best news is that it spares everyone else around you the gory details of your personal drama. At the same time, you're making great headway in your own self-work and your physical health.

The important message to convey to you, especially in the case of old, lingering anger and grudges, is that the ultimate goal for deep healing is forgiveness. It's a must-do for the sake of your own health, and a very necessary final step. And I mean not only for the perpetrator who hurt you but also forgiveness for yourself. Yourself for staying plugged into the negative feelings around the issue. This is one of the beautiful reasons why this technique is called "emotional freedom." Forgiveness is the number one key to unlock the energetic shackles that kept you and the other person bound together living in the past. Said best in an old French proverb, "He has not escaped who drags his chains."

As far as emotional and physical homeostasis is concerned, letting go on a cellular level means you win. Forgiving someone with every fiber of your being with all your heart means that love trumps hate. Remember, the person you hate can't actually feel your hatred, only you do, and you pay for it dearly health-wise. How fair is that?

CHAPTER THIRTY-THREE

Controlling the Unacceptable

The issue of control deserves two chapters in this book because it's a gigantic issue, and I have a lot to say about it. For one thing, absolutely everyone has a control problem in one way or another. ESPECIALLY if you have a serious illness or a secret about your personal life that you feel will destroy family unity and your sense of security.

For certain people, unfortunately, it is the deepest and darkest of all secrets: their sexual preference.

This story is near and dear to my heart and in honor of all my gay Flight Attendant "boyfriends" back in the early 70's. They livened up our flights and kept me on my toes laughing with our quick-witted banter. I got to know my favorites very well. On long, late night flights after our inflight service, it was our time to chill, download, and get real. It was there that my small town world expanded, beginning with a primary course in "Gay 101."

Time and again, they spoke of parental and family rejection. Only the brave ones with a "plan B" had the nerve to cast their fate to the winds and come out to their parents. Over half were shunned, shamed, and rejected by their immediate family after either being discovered or for coming out on their own. Mother/female idolization was far more prevalent when there was father rejection and vice versa.

Enlightened by personal stories, I had a better understanding of what they were up against in this world as human beings. Regardless of their personal challenges, as Flight Attendants, we were a close-knit family of friends. It was a safe environment as a workplace, with lots of love, acceptance, and emotional support.

Here's what I learned in the process. The LGBTQ's born in the era of the "Silent Generation" (1925-1945) versus being born a "Baby Boomer," (1946-1964) had a different set of freedom issues. It made all the difference in who was going to come out, and who never would. It was definitely a generational thing.

The silent generation's fears of discovery, judgment, and persecution were far more intense. The baby boomers, on the other hand, had more leeway due to the cultural revolution of the 60's. Thanks to our pop-culture, people were encouraged to be courageous in their personal expressions.

As a well seasoned EFT practitioner, I've had the opportunity to work with both gay men and women from the silent generation. I have a better understanding of where they've been, how it must feel, and the origin of issues that are currently holding them back health-wise.

It's important to convey this is not my generalization of what the entire LGBTQ community is currently feeling. This is an example of how EFT can help free the fear and suffering of the hurt, closeted, and disenfranchised.

Back in the 50's and early 60's a standard "must have" for every household was to have a "Medical Book." There in plain writing "Homosexuality" was listed under "deviant behaviors." Clearly, it was "abnormal" because the American Medical Association said so. Unfortunately, such statements set the moral compass of the time. God forbid if one of your children had "evil and abnormal" urges, there had to be something wrong with them. Being labeled a "queer" had dire consequences, even life-threatening, in the early years.

It took the American Psychiatric Association until 1973 to change their tune. They removed "Homosexuality" off of their official list of "Mental Disorders." But negative generational opinions of the LGBTQ population had already been set in place.

Through better education and public awareness, things are changing. I'm so glad to know there are more parents who love their LGBTQ children no matter what. You see glimpses of it on Facebook with teens coming out to their parents in videos. They are more likely to become confident adults without all the rejection issues clouding up their lives.

Further, I've been able to witness firsthand, from mom's Spanish/Mexican side of the family, two contrasting examples of gay pride, and gay shame. For more cultural understanding it's important to mention Catholicism is huge for them. Also, in Latin families, especially over 40 years ago, the first born son is supposed to marry, give them grandchildren, and keep the family name alive. When you come from a "good family" and are raised properly, daughters are supposed to dress and act like ladies. They don't act like tomboys, nor do they hang around with other tomboys, it looks bad for the family. You're supposed to be chaperoned while being courted so you can get married and have children. That was the goal. Any deviations to those cultural expectations were a huge disappointment.....and a family embarrassment.

One cousin was raised by parents who loved and supported him unconditionally. His parents had a loving relationship and a happy marriage. Mom stayed home with the kids, and dad worked to bring home the bacon. When my cousin came out to them, he wasn't judged, shamed, or controlled and made guilty by their religious and cultural beliefs. They were proud of their first born son for the person he was, and that didn't change. He was still the same loving, intelligent, funny, artistic and sensitive child they always knew. He had their full support, and they loved and accepted his friends as well. He grew up to be a confident and successful professional in his field of work with a college degree. After 25 years together, he is happily married to the love of his life.

My other two cousins, a brother and sister, were less fortunate. There were other disadvantages that complicated growing up in their home. Their father suffered from PTSD after a catastrophic accident in WW2. God rest his soul, he self-medicated with alcohol and had a very bad problem with it his whole life. What little money he made was spent in the bars after work. Lack of spousal support for household funds kept his wife stressed out, angry and ashamed of her husband, and of herself. Her parents, brothers, and sisters helped them as much as they could, and that added to more shame. Having two gay children on top of everything else absolutely unacceptable. It was unnatural and sinful in the eyes of the church, and another mark against their family. She would never acknowledge them as gay or accept their significant relationships.

Yet, neither one of my cousins played down their gayness, rather, they leaned into it and stood their ground. Each had their own set of challenges living at home, too many to mention. The point is, each fought against extreme resistance in their own way, on their own terms, loud and proud. Together they forged a very close bond of mutual love, acceptance, and empathy for each other. Even though he had long moved away from home, the brother always made an effort to appease and spoil his mother. His sister, still a respectful and dutiful daughter, was far less concerned with placating her. That would involve turning "straight" and dating men. Ah, nope.

By the time the brother received his HIV diagnosis, his father was terminally ill with advanced liver disease. In his typical selfless, considerate style, he chose to spare everyone the news and not add to their worry. He suffered alone in silence with his health condition.

After no-showing a planned visit with his sister, he was discovered ill at his home. He was hospitalized and treated for a ruptured appendix. While recovering from surgery, they discovered a surgical tool left inside his abdominal cavity.

Undergoing a second surgery, he assured his sister that he was okay and to stop worrying. He made her promise to not cancel her scheduled trip to Brazil for work. She would pick him up from the hospital when she returned, and take him home with her to care for him until he recovered. Pensive and uneasy while in Brazil, she went shopping. After all he'd been through she wanted to spoil him with a beautiful ring as a present. Too distracted to choose one, she went back to her hotel. That's when she got the call...he was gone. Without anyone by his side to comfort him in his final moments, he died alone in his hospital room in Dallas.

He had a great big wonderful personality. He was loving, funny, exuberant, flamboyant, intelligent and talented. In private, he fought his own demons from childhood; he shared his struggles with few. You would never guess he was hurting because he never let his guard down. There are those who would argue that letting go of the pain from your past would negate who you are. You wouldn't be who you are today without it. EFT does not give you amnesia, you can't change what happened to you in the past. But you can change your negative emotional and physical response to it. Taking internal stress levels down positively affects your physical health.

It's been 17 years since he's been gone. With my help, his sister found her way out of the complex maze of grief. The anniversary of his death was what she referred to as her "fall depression." She no longer feels that way about that time of year. She now focuses on the way he lived instead of the way he died. She finds comfort in a lifetime of memories together and lasting impressions of his joy for life.

Through our work together she also uncovered a surprising revelation! It held her back without her consciously realizing it, and it was buried deep. Considering how bold and courageous she was coming out as a teenager, it was especially surprising. Low, and behold, amidst all her pride in being gay, was another part of her that felt gay shame. Who knew? If her own mother couldn't accept her for who she was, deep down, she couldn't be on board with herself either. Bingo! Nothing like real internal congruence I always say!

In fact, somewhere along the way she learned to do her best imitation of her critical mother, and use it on herself. Even though she was born undeniably beautiful, she couldn't see it. It was actually hard for me to hear her own opinion about the way she looked. We cleared out the name-calling and criticisms of the past to diffuse negative body images, self-loathing and low self-worth. And just like that, all areas of her life opened up for the better on their own.....without her controlling the outcome.

By gaining emotional freedom from her past, with new clarity, things go her way without all the effort. Life feels much lighter, and much easier for her, without feeling like she needs to fix everyone she loves. She has a huge family of very close-knit friends and is very happy and content in her life. Ten years ago she married her partner of 33 years in one of the most beautiful and elegant weddings I've ever seen.

In a world evolved, there is no shame, guilt or judgment in being LGBT or Q (gender queer) or for being parents of them. And we're loved and accepted for our entire selves as a person, not judged or persecuted for something as personal as sexuality.

In our reality, as it should be, true love and acceptance begin within the confines of our own heart.

CHAPTER THIRTY-FOUR

Out of Control

I went for years without being able to see how controlling "I" actually was. Growing up, my dad had rage issues. I learned at a very young age how to lighten the mood in our house, in essence, control the environment. It was an old habit that kept me "on duty" to hide my social anxiety. EFT collapsed those old stories and changed my life. I now feel relaxed and comfortable being myself in any social situation. It feels wonderful I might add. And that's the point; when you're relaxed with yourself, you're relaxed around other people. Vibing that energy, people tend to feel at ease around you, too.

The issue of feeling "Out of Control" to use an analogy, is like a "tabletop." The "legs" of the table are your supporting life events that hold up the table top. It's your job to systematically kick out each of those legs one by one and collapse that table!

The need for control stems from past events when you felt out of control. It could be your role was being the victim, and you had control taken away from you? Or you were the perpetrator and took control away from someone else? Either way, there you were, out of control.

I've supplied you with a list of possibilities to help recognize yourself. It's a good idea to write down the ones that resonate. And then write down a list of specific events you think made you feel that way. Not the entire story, give each memory a small title that encompasses the entire story. Include the times when you only felt "sort of" out of control too. Everything counts and has an intensity level even if it's a small one.

Okay, here goes, I told you it's a HUGE complexed topic!

WHEN DREAD GETS IN THE WAY (You might be a control freak.)

I call this "The Dread Factor" on my website. [11] I'm speaking to those of you who had used EFT before and dropped out because you just plain dread tapping. You know it works, you've done it, but you won't do it, you put it off, and find reasons not to. It seems to be inconvenient when you do think about it, so you put it off until later, but you never find the time. There's a reason you won't go there, and for your own sake, it's well worth exploring.

Another reason to dread EFT is that it annoys you to give time or power to a certain person or a situation in your past. You're "tired" of thinking about it so you won't go there, you don't see the point.

I can relate to this reason. It could be you feel you've already done your work with cognitive behavioral therapy, and you feel it's behind you. You prefer to work on current issues, ones that feel relevant to you now. I've got news for you, it's worth testing to see if it's actually out of your deeper energy centers. You won't get anywhere without addressing these issues too. Sorry, but it's true, your body isn't done with it. See for yourself and go over them again.

Below, I'll point out the behavioral symptoms of control. In our next book, "Mind-Body Renewal," I'll detail the physical symptoms of control and what to look for. Looking through the list below keep in mind these could be "hidden" control issues. So if you momentarily get stuck on one that "kind of" resonates, write it down it and test for yourself.

CONTROL BY MANIPULATING LOVE
AND COMFORT RESPONSES
(Who loves ya baby?)

This is a huge topic. Here are some common examples for you to pick through to see if you recognize yourself?

Hypochondriasis (you're a hypochondriac)
Doctor hopping, healthcare technique hopping

---

[11] See https://EFTOne.com

Addiction to surgeries
Addicted to drama
Addiction to medical procedures
Over-medicating
Under medicating
Over-focused on physical symptoms, you're pre-occupied by health
concerns and worries
Common interactions with other people involve reporting your
symptoms or pain levels
Seek pity because it feels like someone cares.
You're a people pleaser, a flatterer, you ingratiate (play up to people
for approval so they'll like you)
You're dependent on your relationships
You're always the one who's victimized; it always seems like people
single you out and pick on you
You're needy in relationships
You like being rescued, you need to be saved,
You need to rescue, you like to save.
Hello, co-dependency.

REASONS FOR OVER-CONTROLLING BEHAVIOR
(I won't ever let that happen again!)

Rage-aholic parent/parents
Alcoholic parent/parents,
Drug addicted parent/parents,
Saw parental fighting, physical abuse
Saw sibling emotional/physical abuse
Experienced emotional/physical abuse by a sibling
Experienced childhood physical/emotional abuse
Neglected as a child
You were abandoned by a parent/parents
Schizophrenic/bipolar/personality disorder parent/parents
You're a child of a divorce
You were in foster care
You were adopted

You were molested

You were raped

You have a history of one or more childhood surgeries and
hospitalizations

You have a history of serious childhood illness and hospitalizations

TELLTALE CONTROLLING BEHAVIOURS
(Enough about me, let's talk about you. What do you think of me?)

You ingratiate people, (play-up to them) giving gratuitous
compliments so they'll "like" you

Elicit (fish for) compliments

Jealous natured

You manipulate things to go your way

Moody

You sulk even on happy occasions

Your moods dominate

You're an insomniac

Everything has to be perfect

You have to be perfect

You can't let go of anything material

You can't let go of anything emotional

Only you know best

You don't trust anyone else's decisions

You want everyone to go along with you

You get angry or frustrated or throw a fit if things don't go your way.

You have a dominating or bossy personality

Your campaign about how good you are to other people

You think everyone should cater to your wants and needs on your
terms

You dominate conversations

You're a bad listener

You're talking inside your head when someone else is talking to you

You only wait for opportunities talk again in a conversation

You interrupt and talk over others

You're more interesting, important, smarter

You know it all
Everyone else is wrong
Everything should be based on your decision
Your level of expectations must be met or you become deeply
    disappointed, angry and frustrated
No one can do it better than you
You become ill when you don't receive enough attention
You've lied about an illness or disease to receive attention
You know people in your life who are "pushovers," and you take
    advantage
You use people and feel superior about it
You feel helpless become destructive if you can't control a situation
Road rage feels normal
You have physically hurt someone out of frustration when things
    haven't gone your way
You verbally or physically threaten children, spouse or loved one if
    you don't get what you want.

I Accept Myself

What it all boils down to is Self Acceptance. It's so important you're congruent with that. I think it's a separate issue to work through rather than force-feeding the concept.

Traditionally, part of the EFT formula when you're working on a problem is a "setup phrase." You're stating the specific problem, and the self-acceptance statement, you accept yourself in spite of the fact you have an issue.

Generically it sounds like this;

"Even though I have this_______(state the issue)

I deeply and completely love and accept myself."

Before my introduction to EFT, it never occurred to me that it was possible I didn't love and accept myself. After all, intellectually, if I'm proposing to be a well-balanced individual, of course, I do! Uh, not so much.

The truth is, it's hard for a lot of people to say they deeply and completely love and accept themselves. It became very evident the more people I worked with. I've concluded that self-love, and self-acceptance, the lack thereof, was a huge problem. It also came with huge amounts of denial wrapped around it intellectually.

So I came up with a way to bypass it all together by telling yourself the story while you're tapping. I call it "Grumble Tap" and I show you how to do that on my website, EFTOne.com.

In private practice, I use the self-acceptance statement as a way to gauge how my clients feel. Here's how you can test yourself at home alone. Say this out loud; "I deeply and completely love and accept myself." Now put your hand over your heart, close your eyes, and say it out loud again.

Give yourself a moment to see how it feels. Pay attention to what your heart's saying, and not what your head thinks your heart should say. You'll find out exactly where you stand. Is it 100% true? If not, what's the percentage of truth?

If you've said it out loud and it's not feeling 100% true, you've got a Heart Chakra blockage. If it sounds kind of corny or you feel a bit detached to your response, it's still a reflection of the way you feel about yourself. There is something about you that you disagree with and worth investigating. More about that in my next book, but it means blocked to yourself, and more than likely, it's blocking love in other areas of your life as well.

Keep in mind the way you feel about yourself affects the people in your life and how they respond to you. If you're not congruent with self-respect, you're teaching other people how to disrespect you too. Negative personal views also make a difference in the way you interpret other people's reaction to you. That determines how you react to them. It's a negative energetic chain reaction. It's an energy you're vibrating whether you realize it or not. Removing Heart Chakra blockages are good for your heart and the many ways it governs your well being,

No matter what you've been told by a parent or a peer, self-love, and self-acceptance doesn't mean you're conceited or "full of yourself." It means you have a healthy regard for your health and wellbeing. It means you're considerate and kind to yourself and the people you love, and all living things. It means that you have respect for yourself, and you're respectful of others. It's a good thing. So when it comes to self-love and acceptance, you might just be your own biggest problem. That's a real powerful self-discovery at any age.

Knowing the way you really feel should then become your top priority in your self-improvement goals. Gauging your amount of self-love and self-acceptance will be your tip-off for where to go first. Look for past supporting evidence, the reasons why you're unlovable, why you're unacceptable.

When you change your internal attitude about yourself, self-care becomes effortless and justifiable. For example, working out becomes something you look forward to instead of dread. Eating healthier isn't a hassle anymore because you're worth it, and that's just the half of it. All the other things you would love to do for yourself that have been put on the back burner becomes something you can do without over-thinking about it. The positive chain reaction goes straight across the board, too many to mention. Bottom line, you give a damn because you're worth it. It's priceless.

CHAPTER THIRTY-SIX

Ready, Willing and Able

When you're "READY" to commit to your own healing is when you are "WILLING" to view all possible sides of yourself. And you are "ABLE" to do that with focus because you want it.

Control issues are the most common form of self-sabotage. With you in your own way, nothing, not even EFT, will help you reach your health goals and find personal peace. For your own sake, it's well worth the time to test and see if control is one of your blind spots. Before you think that's a big character flaw, we all have blind spots, even me.

If you don't think control is an issue, aren't you even interested to see what's in there for the heck of it? Addressing "possible" control problems is a great test to see if you're in denial.

Example; starting at the karate chop point you might say; "It's hard to admit I have a control problem." Finish the tapping sequence while saying; "Releasing this control problem."

Pay attention to see if you have a relaxation response during your tapping. Look for yawns, sighing, tingling sensations or a light-headed feeling. If it's a yes........you might have a control problem. I'm just sayin.

I get into the physical role of "Chakras" in my next book, but there's something more you should know about how they relate to illnesses. In the case of serious diseases and chronic health problems, the heart chakra is also blocked. That means loving care for yourself is to some degree limited. The amount of heartache you've experienced in the past dictates how bad your love deficit.

The chain reaction to the lack of self-love is a lack of ability to self-nurture. Again, some more so than others. With the scale being unbalanced, you could also over-nurture rather than under-nurture. Stored inside of the heart energy center on a cellular level, lies supporting evidence against yourself and others. Those are the negative events and negative messages in your life that prove to you that you're not "worth" it. It's the stuff you bought into and agree with. And it can be there even if you're not consciously aware of it.

Unworthiness contributes to controlling the amount of help you are willing to accept. Some people may claim in loud voices that they want the help and appear very proactive in their quest.

Yet, impatience with their bodies (anger and distrust in self) keep them from following through in any one therapy. In extreme cases, they stop the treatment as soon as they discover they're actually recovering. They won't allow healing to take place because there is a secondary gain in staying ill. Being "cared for" fills an empty space. This is only one aspect of control and how it's used for self-sabotage.

There are a variety of personal reasons why controlling your surroundings feel safe. Finding the supporting events and diffusing them, will strengthen your immune system. Fear is not a healing energy. Too much of it causes imbalance and keeps your adrenals on hyper-vigilant mode.

CHAPTER THIRTY-SEVEN

Back At Ya!

This next story is a very clever way to override control blockages. Use it if you feel stuck and not getting anywhere in your EFT self-work.

The Boomerang Tapping Technique was developed by EFT practitioner, the late Hypatia Kelly-Butte.

Her technique uses EFT using a "virtual proxy." This allows stepping outside of your control boundaries and tap for yourself "once removed." In essence, you throw it out there like it's coming from someone else, and it comes back to you directly like a boomerang.

This energetic distancing is "guessing" how you think someone else thinks you feel. Since only you know how you feel, you will always correctly guess the intensity of your issues. When you step out of the equation, someone else's interpretation may ultimately be kinder than how you're actually feeling. Confused yet? Lol! It's a great way to begin getting acquainted with your feelings, and finally owning them.

"THE BOOMERANG TAPPING TECHNIQUE" (Tapping by Virtual Proxy)

In loving memory of Hypatia Kelly-Butte. May you bask in the glow of eternal love and light, and your heart recognize unbridled joy throughout eternity. - R.M.

Hypatia was born and raised in New York City. She was the only child of a narcissistic single mother, a Rockette, at Radio City Music Hall. And it was all about her mother all the time. Her clothes, her figure, her hair, her makeup and her boyfriends, while Hypatia's needs came last. Her father left the family and divorced her mother when she was little. Mother went on to marry 7 more times. She was lonely as a small child, left to her own devices to take care of herself while her mother worked and socialized. According to Hypatia; "The woman didn't have a maternal bone in her body."

Hypatia contacted me because she had stage 4 breast cancer. I never shy away from the severity of a disease, including late-stage illnesses. As I've said before, my work many times becomes a deep "emotional hospice." It's a win-win situation getting rid of past regrets and disappointments, old grudges. It lightens the burdens of your soul. The rest is up to a higher power.

Why did she wait so long to get help? In large part, it was because of what I call PROFESSIONAL RESISTANCE - (If I'm so good, why can't I do this myself?)[12]

This is a control issue that stems from low self-esteem, embarrassment, and shame. Common issues that can stand between professionals when seeking help from peers. The typical self-talk would be "If I'm so smart, and I've helped others, why can't I figure this out on my own?"

I've got two words for you. Blind spot.

Hypatia was self-treating with a vegan diet, herbal medicinals, and aroma therapies. She asked for my help in finding her emotional blind spots. From taking her history, the location of her cancer made perfect sense to me. From an energetic standpoint, breast cancer stems from a profound lack of nurturing. She didn't want anything more to do with medical science, and she was done with her doctors. That was her life decision entirely. But she was blackmailed and bullied by the medical professionals for not cooperating with their treatment plan. Unless she followed their recommendations, they refused to help her with palliative care, to ease her pain and discomforts.

---

[12] https://www.dropbox.com/s/3bcnxu32aximq4h/Professional%20Resistance.pdf?dl=0

She had a Harvard degree in Architecture and a degree in Anthropology from UC Berkeley. After having what she called a "spiritual epiphany," Hypatia became an EFT practitioner.

Her name wasn't always Hypatia. She named herself after the great Hellenistic Neoplatonist philosopher, astronomer, and mathematician, Hypatia. As a prominent thinker and wise counselor, Hypatia taught at the Neoplatonic School of Alexandria, Egypt. Because she was Pagan with no plans to convert, the Christians were suspicious of her. Consequently, she was persecuted by false rumors and removed from her professorial position. Hypatia was then attacked and murdered by a mob of Christian monks who tore her body apart and set her on fire. Pretty safe to say she was dead after all that. I bet they even stomped on her smoldering ashes. She died a martyr to ignorance.

But you can't keep a good girl down, so the great and ancient Hypatia is now a twentieth-century feminist icon. Brava Diva!

It was an interesting choice of "new" name for her. It also gave me insight into how she viewed herself as a person, and how she viewed her position in life.

Our treatment goals were for pain management and the expulsion of negative emotions. I never "treat" a disease directly. My focus with clients is helping them to find love, understanding, and forgiveness. These are the healing energies that have the ability to override a disease like cancer. A metaphor for cancer could be "what's eating you?" Get it?

Our initial sessions helped her to "own" her feelings and untangle the giant knot of rage around her mother. Pain relief was immediate and was a pleasant benefit. She began to feel clear-headed again and started back to writing after a long hiatus of feeling stuck. After one of our sessions, Hypatia emailed me to say; "It is so apparent to me that there are no trivial memories. Everything is a chord back into the center. Love Hypatia." I agree with her completely.

Hypatia was a proud and active member of Rue Hass's (one of the early EFT Masters) mentoring program. Rue chose her to be a presenter at an upcoming "Tapper's Gathering." She was set to introduce her new tapping technique, "Boomerang Tapping." She was very excited by this new boost to her career. We worked to help her feel strong enough to make the trip. She exited this world before it could ever happen.

In honor of Hypatia, I am pleased to pay it forward and present her creative twist on surrogate tapping.

In her words:

"The Boomerang Tapping Technique expands on the power of surrogate tapping. I believe that by tapping as another person and giving them the true words of feelings held, a field of compassion opens up. The potential for deep understanding broadens, and true sharing of the release of misunderstanding can be realized by all".

I see this technique as an energetic form of role-playing. For one thing, it has the potential to be a very powerful relationship tool. Marriage and family councilors who use EFT could incorporate it in couples sessions. The applications of boomeranging are limitless.

To the best of my ability, I will describe my knowledge and understanding of how to use it.

Surrogate tapping is imagining you are the person of your intention. It's you tuning into them. You tap for their issues as if they were yours.

Hypatia described her technique as "reverse surrogate tapping." This means tapping as if you were someone else surrogate tapping for you. You twice removed. Is that far enough away for some of you? Lol!

Boomerang tapping is useful for addressing certain "parts" of ourselves that can't see that we can't speak our truth. It's also a large part of the way "people helpers" feel. They are more comfortable helping other people before themselves. The origin of this type of self-sabotage is usually limited beliefs about being a "good person." I'm guessing it's a family myth for most.

Hypatia's initial discovery for throwing her emotions somewhere else came out of an exasperating moment. She was stuck working on herself after several rounds of tapping. So she threw the problem at her dog, Ruga, to speak for her, since she felt her dog knew her heart. Ruga had just given her that "you are my most beloved person in the world" look with her expressive eyes. If you're an animal lover, you know the look, and you know that to be true.

As with surrogate tapping, she mentally stepped behind Ruga's eyes, "becoming" her dog. She could see herself as she imagined Ruga saw her. With energetic distancing, to her surprise, she quickly collapsed her issue!

Her set-up phrase: "I'm Ruga, and even though my mom is sad, she is the most loved person in the world right now, by me." Reminder Phrase; "I love mom more than anything else in this world."

According to Hypatia, the SUDs (subjective units of distress) plummeted to complete diffusion. She called it "magic," and when it happens to you, it's a good way to describe it!

In essence, she sent herself the love and acceptance she needed through her dog. Sad isn't it? It's the love that she couldn't connect with emotionally. At least I think that's part of what happened.

Although this may seem as simply surrogate tapping, it appears to be the double entendre. This type of energetic manipulation comes back as your own. EFT founder called this "borrowing benefits." It seems to be the differentiating factor. It is worthy of further experimentation. Boomerang...be prepared to accept the gift when it returns to you.

Curious addendum:

Hypatia was a "Vedic" astrologer, the current name for ancient "Hindu" astrology. Western astrology focuses on the sun and the planets against the backdrop of the stars. Vedic astrology focuses on the stars themselves and has different interpretations and predictions.

Hypatia told me about a prediction given her by her mentor, a renowned Vedic Astrologer. She told me it was considered unethical to do so, but he foretold the time of her death and the year it would happen. She never shared with me when that would be.

Knowing nothing about Vedic astrology, I strongly disagreed. And I offered my same opinion about the power of suggestion. It's like terminally ill patients buying into their doctor's prognosis and lasting as exactly long as they're told they would. Did she die on someone else's schedule? Only she knows that now.

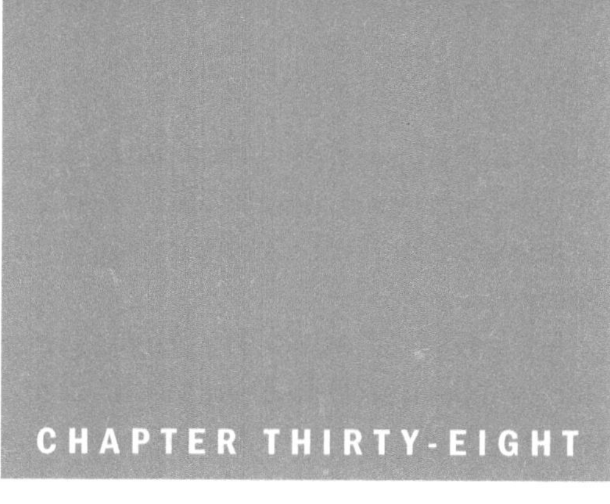

The Vanishing Twin

Throughout the book, I've given you examples of the broad range of applications of EFT. Here's an unusual story, and for me, one that completely registered new realizations. It's about the validity of prenatal emotional responses when life begins. Do events in utero really add to our emotions once we're born? Is this yet another layer of emotions to pay attention to and deal with? Seriously, are you kidding me? Uh, yeah.

This is a story about prenatal trauma and fetal emotions. Before this experience, I didn't think stuff like this could happen. After this experience, beyond a shadow of a doubt, it's cellular realness.

I was at my tia and tio's 50th wedding-anniversary party in El Paso, Texas, where I met this young couple. They heard about tapping and wondered if I could help their two-year-old son, Stephen. His behavior was an enigma to everyone, and of great concern to both of them.

Although we were at a party, they wanted to know more about EFT. I love to talk about it so invited them to a quick trial run of what it looked like, and how it felt. They agreed, and off we went to my uncle's private office with their son.

For a young boy with inexplicable behavioral problems, I asked her about her pregnancy. She said she was sick for weeks before she found out she was pregnant. Later, sonogram results showed two separate placentas. One fetus, a boy, was thriving, while the other, a girl, appeared much smaller in comparison, and was no longer alive. The clinical name for this is the "Vanishing Twin Syndrome." She said she wasn't emotional about the loss of the infant whatsoever. It was a tough pregnancy, and for the next four months she was nauseated every day. She couldn't tolerate smells and scents of anything without an extreme hypersensitive reaction.

The baby boy delivered at 33 weeks. He weighed in at only 4 pounds, and from the size of his diminished umbilical cord, malnourished. Before long he was finally able to leave the neonatal unit and able to go home. For the next six months, everyone enjoyed the peaceful, happy infant. He slept throughout the night without disruption. And then things drastically changed.

After his first six-months round of vaccinations, the baby ran a fever for six days. Concerned, the parents questioned the pediatrician about the prolonged fever. The doctor told them it was "coincidental" and he was "fighting a virus." He denied the shots had anything to do with it. All the parents knew was that he wasn't the same baby after those shots.

When the fever finally subsided, Stephan changed into a moody, irritable, difficult baby. He would wake up three to four times a night crying inconsolably. As he grew older (1-2yrs) he threw terrible temper tantrums. It happened so often, and he was so out of control, his parents were exasperated. With no other course of action to distract him, they would stand with him fully clothed in a cold shower to shock him out of it.

The parents noticed his extreme discomfort in large crowds. If it was noisy, bright, and filled with movement, he couldn't handle it. The slightest change in his immediate environment would be enough to make him hysterical. It could happen if they were out socially with his family, or if he awoke to a visiting houseguest after napping. He would become "over-stimulated" around other children, and angered by their unwanted attention. It made it tough for his mom to pick up the older children from school because he had to ride along with her.

It was especially hard to see how much anger and hostility he had toward his older brother and father. He'd throw a fit if they tried to hug, touch, or sometimes even look at him. In fact, the only time the dad got a kiss from his little son was when he was leaving to go to work. They believe it's because he was happy to see him leave.

The boy will be three years of age this July but only began speaking within the last six months. When the mother told the Pediatrician that she suspected he was autistic, he was non-committal. But he did assign him to Early Childhood Intervention caseworkers. He also wrote a prescription for Occupational Therapy to deal with "sensory issues."

Well, the shots were the obvious problem with him. But I was more interested in the "pink elephant" in the room no one was talking about. The fact was he began his life with his twin sister. He felt her in distress and felt her die right next to him, up close. The energy of her presence remained as she deteriorated alongside him until he was delivered. He never felt her again.

I explained surrogate tapping to them. Imagine themselves being him, in utero, see through his eyes, and tap like it's him doing it. The little boy was becoming restless and wanted to leave the room. I stepped the session into high gear!

"I'm Stephan, even though I'm lost without her, I'm a good boy, and mommy, and daddy misses her too." "I'm lost without her, I don't know where she is, we all miss her."

After our first round of tapping Stephan relaxed, yawned, advanced toward his father. We were stunned when he proceeded to drape himself over his father's lap.

From the tapping, the mother realized that no matter how brief, her daughter's life did count. And she mattered, especially to her twin. Perhaps some of his "acting out" was the residue from the change?

The second round of tapping was; "'Even though I'm afraid and I'm mad she's not here, I'm a real good boy, and I'll try and have fun now."

Reminder Phrase: "I'm so mad she's not here; I don't like it without her."

The third and last round of tapping was to acknowledge his feelings of loss and honor the fact she once lived.

"Even though I'm sad that you're gone, I'm a really good boy, and I'm glad you were with me."

Reminder Phrase: "I'm so sad that you're gone, I'm glad you were with me, I'll never forget you as long as I live, sending love to my sister."

All three of them felt relaxed and peaceful afterward. Stephan calmly asked to leave the room to go play. We returned to the party without knowing what to expect. How could something so "far out" as prenatal EFT work on such a complicated problem?

And yet, without much fanfare, we saw Stephan running past us laughing with the other kids. To their surprise, he was engaging in physical contact! The mom came up to me and said; "Did you see that"? We agreed not to make a big deal about it but continued to be stunned by his actions for the rest of the evening. His entire family including his grandparents noticed a profound change in his attitude.

It used to be that Stephan would dictate the time to go home when he'd had enough. But this time the whole family stayed at the anniversary party as long as everyone else did. The coolest thing yet was that he was volunteering kisses and hugs to anyone who wanted them--including a gigantic kiss and very tight hug for me!

I left El Paso two days later, but the changes in his behavior continued to unfold for weeks afterward. According to his delighted parents, Stephan is much more pleasant to be with in general. Other family members and friends have noticed that they can see a big difference in him. He seems much calmer. In fact, on his last evaluation, his E.C.I. caseworker determined she wasn't needed anymore!

Behavioral modifications per his parents went as follows:

He has not thrown a temper tantrum since the tapping, and his anger subsided "substantially."

It seems that he's developed a sense of humor! His sister and brother get a kick out of how funny he is, and his animated antics have them laughing all the time.

The picking up the kids at school nightmare doesn't happen anymore. Now he loves that time of day and interacts with all kids.

For the first time ever, the whole family can stay in the church for the duration of the mass without incident. He even holds hands for the Lords Prayer!

And best of all is the change with his father. Stephan now looks forward to being with him, spending most of the day with him without protest if mom steps out for errands.

If ever there is a moment even slightly reminiscent of an old tantrum, they have him tap on his karate chop point or his crown, and he snaps right out of it!

It still rocks my world to see this young boy thrive. Whether he remembers it or not, I can tell there is a knowing. In a crowd full of people, he still makes it a point to run up to me and give me a huge hug and a kiss! I never turn it down.

Bloody Murder

Okay, we're down to talking about unfortunate events in everyday life that can happen. What if you saw something you wish you hadn't? Is it important to remember the way someone died so you'll never forget? Or is it more important to remember how someone lived and see <u>that</u> in your mind's eye instead? This article is about a horrific traumatic event that stunted the life of a witness. He couldn't stop seeing it in his mind's eye for many years afterward.

When a negative event occurs, it's encoded by a special group of molecules called the neuropeptides. They live in the past and keep you there too. You can call them up whenever you want to; they have a good memory. That's why you can mentally bring up physical sensations from an emotional event just like it was yesterday. Not only that, it's also not healthy for you to keep them ruminating around.

Using EFT to work on a traumatic event will not erase the fact that it happened. It frees you from feeling the negative physical and emotional response to it. Who needs to hang onto toxic waste?

Witnessing a murder is a specific traumatic event that produces post-traumatic stress. It's one specific traumatic event as your main focus vs. soldiers in combat who can experience more than one, more than once. In this story, you'll see how many facets just one event can have. That's why it's important to ask the help of an EFT professional to get you through it as quickly and as painlessly as possible.

Years ago I was so excited to tell everyone about how well EFT works, I wanted everyone to know about it. But not everyone wanted to listen, especially my family and friends, I had to tone it down a bit. In hindsight, I probably was scaring them. I'm sure they thought I went off the deep end for a while! Lol!

Once I understood that self-help is a personal path to discover on your own when you're ready, I chilled about it. So it was cool when my friend, Freeman, asked "me" for some help and not the other way around.

I remember once in conversation he said his right and left brain felt blocked. His love for music (he plays guitar) was uninspired, and he didn't feel like "tackling" math equations like he used to (he's a mathematician). I figured, okay, he's stuck for some reason. I didn't know it then, but Freeman witnessed an armed robbery and a murder in a restaurant in El Paso, Texas 18 years ago.

Months later he attended one of my introductory lectures about EFT. It took the mystery out of what I do, which led him to ask me for help. I'm so glad he did.

He sat down in the chair in my office and said, "I saw a murder, and I'm ready to let this go now. It was a random act of violence, and I just happened to be there."

I have my PTSD clients fill out a standard questionnaire form for PTSD. I use it as a tracking device for levels of distress. As a follow-up, I have them fill out the same form within a few months to compare and check for any lingering aspects. Showing the client the changes between the two leaves little room for doubt.

The levels of distress are from 0-5 on the PTSD checklist. He had a 2 level of repeated, disturbing memories. 3 level disturbing dreams, 2 level at reliving it, and moderate physical reactions with subtle reminders of the event. It was a 4 level at thinking or talking about it. 2 level avoiding activities that remind him of the event, and no trouble at all remembering the details of the event. He had a moderate loss of interest in things he used to enjoy and felt distant from other people. Irritability, angry outbursts, difficulty concentrating were at a 2. So was feeling on guard, and being easily startled, a level 2.

For Freeman's first EFT experience I gave him tapping instructions and asked him to pay attention to any physical sensations in his body. Also to look for physical relaxation responses, like yawning, sighing, belching. It's a sure sign of energy movement. In first time sessions with newbies, there's always so much going on at once that's new to them, I help them sort it out. I'll call it to their attention when they yawn or sigh in case they didn't notice.

Men, in general, tend to play down their reactions and emotions. I offered him a round of tapping beforehand to defuse the intensity of the memory and make it easier for him. But he assured me that we didn't need to sidestep because it happened a long time ago, and it didn't feel as intense as it used to be. I wasn't buying it and started our session with "The Tearless Trauma Technique" aka therapeutic dissociation.

I asked him not to step into the event yet, don't look at it. Stand alongside of it without looking and give it a small title to encompass the memory. Without looking at the memory, if he could, guess the intensity. For a memory that big, according to him it was a low intensity 1 or a 2. His best guess without looking.

He titled it "The Day of Change."

"I can accept myself, even though I had this Day of Change." Immediately, I noticed facial flushing, rapid breathing, and a light sweat on his face. We kept tapping until that subsided. He then felt a heaviness-type feeling in his chest, so we tapped for "this feeling in my chest" until it went away. Again, checking for guessed intensity levels until he felt certain it was low.

My first approach to this memory is as if it's a movie, in EFT called the "Movie Technique." If it was a movie, how long would it last? In all, Freeman said the movie took about a minute to run through in his mind. We tapped through it in his mind, in order, starting from the beginning. Clip by clip, we collapsed the intensities from the prelude to the aftermath. He was ready to test and see if there was anything left. I had him tell the story.

"I walked up to the register to pay my friend working at his family's restaurant." I made him stop right there, and asked him to give what happens next a small title. He called it "pandemonium." As soon as he said the word pandemonium, he lost it and covered his face with his hands, overcome with emotion.

I took one of his hands and tapped on his fingers, gamut point, and other points away from his face until the wave of emotion went away. Calm enough to narrate, he told me exactly what "pandemonium" meant.

In his words:

"The doors flew open and two men with guns came charging in; instinctively, we all held our hands up. I heard gunshots and heard a bullet fly past my ear, and saw my friend, Tommy, fall to the floor. Everyone scattered and people were overturning tables, screaming, and ducking for cover. I was the only one who stayed with Tommy."

"I laid him across my lap and tried to find where he was bleeding. I found a bullet hole under his armpit, and put my fingers inside the wound to try to stop the bleeding."

"Do you know what blood smells like? I can still smell the blood. I still remember the shock of seeing that much blood. I can still feel the blood flowing through my fingers. I can still feel his pulse weakening; I felt his life slipping away. I was helpless to stop it because the wound was so severe. My friend died in my lap."

He was able to tell and see the story from a distance for the first time. And he could do it without squashing down the sadness. "Is that unusual for you?" I asked. He said; "Yes, it's not how it usually goes. I'm a wreak for a week after I let myself see it again."

But he was still angry at the "situation" since, according to Freeman, it was a random act of violence. What really pissed him off was that his friend's own family stayed hidden and didn't go to his aid. He got his power back on all counts using my "Bitch Tap Method™". He bitched out loud about the unfairness of the situation, and at the "cowards" who saved their own necks and chose not to help.

Prematurely on purpose, I offered a pre-frame just to see where we were at. I said; "You know, it's a place of honor to be there at the time to comfort someone who's dying, especially a friend."

He said, "No, it was awful. I don't know why it happened to me."

For our last round of tapping, I started off by using his words and reframed the final event. "Even though it was awful, I don't know why it happened to me, what's true is, if not for me, Tommy would have bled to death alone. So even though I risked my life, and it scared the shit out of me to be there for him, I was a friend to him until the end."

Boom! The cognitive shift was immediate. The "alternate" way to look at it collapsed the old belief right at the karate chop point!

"That's true! I'm glad I was there to comfort him. Maybe it wasn't such a random act, after all? It was his time to die, and his way to exit. I was supposed to be there for him because it set off a major change of events in my life for the better."

"Because of Tommy I stopped doing what other people expected of me and followed my own dreams. At least he died fast, that's the best anyone can hope for."

He was completely relaxed when he left the session, saying he was going to go home and take a nap. What's amazing is how 18 years of pain dissolved in less than an hour. And his energies kept right on shifting after that day.

In a one-month follow-up, he was excited to be working on the advanced math equations he didn't feel like "tackling" before! He's back to playing guitar, writing music, and learning traditional songs for his repertoire. He said he felt much lighter, more energetic than he can ever remember. And didn't dream the "old clips" from the event anymore. "Is that unusual?" I asked; he said, "Absolutely!"

Eight weeks later, his comparison PTSD questionnaire is outstanding. All but two questions about trouble falling asleep and feeling irritable were answered with a 2 meaning "a little bit." This suggests other emotional issues yet addressed. The remaining questions were answered: "none at all."

Nevertheless, his impression of his first and only EFT experience, in his words: "It's like letting go of your suitcase after a very long trek. You fall into complete relaxation and relief."

To this day, occasionally when we get together, not every time, I'll ask him if it ever crosses his mind? His answer remains a resounding no, never.

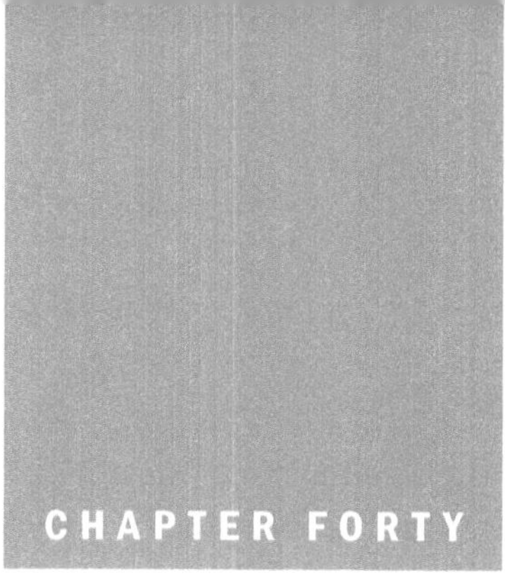

What's More...

You can never have enough personal peace, that's why I'm so passionate about teaching you how to do it yourself! On the instructional portion of our website, after you learn the basics, you can test your knowledge with the mini quizzes at the end of each lesson.

The next thing for you to explore and learn is how to use "EVERYDAY EFT." Use it for everyday issues, and believe me, there's a lot of stuff to work on out there, I can't begin to mention them all!

Take me for example. Remember my childhood Chiropractic drama story? It's pretty safe to assume that I was absolutely terrified of office visits to our family doctor. My experiences can help you get over your fears of medical procedures including pre-surgical fear, dental office phobias.

My first-hand experience with every phase of this process will help you to untangle your fears in detail. With anxiety removed, you'll be able to willingly accept the help of medical professionals for your own good.

For your benefit, I'll go into detail. I'll illustrate the different layers of a phobia, (sights, sounds, smells, physical feelings). It's the type of detail you need to look for and acknowledge (own) to completely collapse your phobia.

My mom always took good care of us holistically, thank goodness, so it wasn't very often I was required to see the doctor. But every single time I went it always seemed to involve a dog-gone stinking shot! I don't mind saying, it always fricken hurt like bloody hell and stung my skin like a wasp bite.

The truth be known, my fears began back at the house just being told I had a doctor's appointment. The feeling in my stomach felt like butterflies jumping off a cliff. I'd become very quiet, hoping she wouldn't notice me and forget the appointment. In the car, driving closer to the office was okay until we got to the side of town where his office was located. By then, the anxiety in my stomach was so over the top I wanted to throw up.

Once the car was parked, my eyes would begin to form tears. Walking through the front door, I got hit with the scary smell of isopropyl alcohol. Next was the nurse at the front desk in a crisp, starched white uniform dress and nurse's cap. When the door shut behind me, I was officially trapped.

I'd start my crying in earnest in the waiting room, wailing and making a big commotion, my mom tried her best to politely shut me up.

Then finally, the moment I dreaded the very most, was when my name was called gave me that sinking feeling in my gut, as the nurse came to get us. This meant I had to be pushed through the door and forced to sit on the examination table.

Once I finished scanning the room for instruments of torture that could cause me pain, there was that precious, sweet moment of reprieve...the wait. We waited because he was busy, so for me, every moment without him counted as a good thing.

Finally, the door would swing open with the force of authority, and there he stood, shiny-skinned, dour-faced, and unsmiling. Wearing a long starched white coat, and a shiny silver stethoscope hanging off his neck, he would size me up with his eyes while my mom narrated.

With no time for niceties, before I knew it, he was all up in my personal space without apology, inspecting me like a 4H farm animal. The terrible moment when he turned his back to us meant that he was buttering up his 20-foot needle attached to a great, big, giant glass syringe. As he walked toward me, he'd make the fluid squirt out of the needle to remove the air bubble, and that's when I would start to panic and begin screaming.

The nurse would come in and she and my mom would have to hold me down as he administered the damn shot while I writhed and screamed at the top of my lungs. I remember it stinging so badly, it actually made me more angry than frightened. So now I'd scream because I was pissed off that it hurt, but also, it meant I lost (over-powered), and they won.

Believe me, this experience was so bad, if I had the choice, it wouldn't matter if my bloody limb was dangling from my body by a thread of tissue. I would still deny anything was ever wrong with me so I wouldn't have to go to his office.

All those emotions, the fear, and anxiety, the histrionics, the stress I put myself through was simply because I was afraid of needles. Okay, the glass syringe was a close second. That was it. How much do you want to bet if I weren't so afraid, that shot wouldn't have hurt as much? If I weren't so pissed off that they managed to shove that needle into my skin, it wouldn't have stung so much?

I can laugh now, but as a small child, I managed to turn a simple office procedure into a Spanish Inquisition torture scene, stressing everyone out. If we knew about EFT back then, this would have been a non-issue entirely.

Dealing with "Medical Procedures" (including dental visits) is something everyone should have in their "EFT Back Pocket." And after surgical procedures, there's "Post-surgical pain management and healing." It's an actual "do it yourself" adjunctive healing tool to manage your post-surgical pain and discomfort naturally. In doing so, you'll actually speed up the time it takes for you to heal. For one thing, it helps to remove limiting beliefs around your prognostic outcome. Negative thoughts and thinking can come at you from many different angles. It could be anything from a horror story about someone who had the same surgery, or maybe your doctor predicts it's going to be a long, painful healing process. It's worth trying EFT to find out for yourself how effective it is.

The value of learning how to use EFT for everyday issues is that it makes your life much easier. If you clear the path, making room for more joy and happiness, you also pass it along energetically without even trying, and that's a good thing. Less moody and angry, more patience and love, exactly what the world needs now.

There is so much to teach you, so on my website I've covered a lot of topics on audio. There are also funny little illustrations (my personality kinda comes through!) of how to apply EFT to a variety of everyday things.

I cover "Relationship Issues" and show you how to find and turn off the real reasons why you're accepting or giving verbal abuse. I show you how to get your mojo back from unfaithful mates, and how to untangle that web of deceit. How to get over breakups or divorce and grow, how to move forward without regrets.

There's a section on "Friends and Enemies" and how to accept, understand, forgive, or release toxic relationships with love. Guilt-free.

You'll learn about "Money Matters" and the ways money can seem like the enemy at both ends of the spectrum. I'll show you how diffuse the underlying emotional causes for the "lack" mentality, and get to the reasons for under-spending.

For many, a bigger problem (than being a tight-wad!) with money is over-spending, anxiety shopping, and massive credit card debt. These are all sugar-coated methods of self-sabotage that come back to bite you in the ass when reality sets in. With diligence, tapping to work on the emotional drivers of over-spending (anxiety) will allow you to get ahold of yourself and stop the madness pronto!

"General Work Place Stressors" for different professions including people helpers who deal with trauma, or for those who are challenged by a daily coworker "attitude" while at work. I listed the more common types (not including Base Jumpers and the like) of professions to give you examples of the variety of stresses there are at work.

If you're a people helper (i.e., doctor or first responder), it's not uncommon to feel like there are other people who have it worse than you do because you see so many bad things. Your needs are still important, and you'll learn how to feel entitled to them, and worthy of the time it takes to help yourself. Bottom line, if you're not in a good state of emotional and physical health, you're not vibing the nurturing, healing energy you need to help others as well.

If it's a different type of work stress like bad bosses, bullies, or project performance anxiety, to name a few, you'll learn how to navigate your day fluidly, and find your worry-free center after work.

Certainly, you can tailor any of my specific examples on my website to anything you do for a living, for your specific type of job stress. Your goal is to learn how to shake off your day energetically to feel centered and balanced. Without all the workday distractions you'll heighten your appreciation for your precious life at home. And your private retreat should be peaceful, you deserve it.

"Event Stressors" - a big topic, but to name a few of the more common:

Weddings, with all the trimmings, like bridezillas, diva mothers-in-law, and who's walking whom down the aisle. Why plug into other people's need for drama and give anyone the power to take away your special day? If you're the bridezilla, you can learn how to check yourself, and find balance in your anticipation for the big event.

Family reunion stress (especially if you're Hispanic!) Bar/Bat Mitzvahs, anniversary parties, and holiday party dread. You might hear "Your weight is up," or if you lost weight, "You're too skinny, you look like a toothpick." The anticipation of judgments, criticisms, grudges, and so forth can cause you to brace for impact long before you even attend the event. You'll learn how to relax the social anxiety, and feel comfortable in your own skin. Relaxed energy is just as conspicuous as feeling on guard and ready for attack.

Road Rage has specific emotional drivers (reasons) which require working on more than one emotion to defuse them, and it's not just anger. I show you how to retrace the tentacles of your feelings so you can break it down to the core level. Once you turn off those negative power switches, there's "peace in the valley," and driving turns into a zen experience for you and not a "Roller Ball" tournament. You'll feel a deep sense of relief. Your goal is to own it, release it, forgive yourself for your shortcomings, forgive the "perpetrator" and move on. It's pretty simple. By the way, have I mentioned before that resolution is great for your health?

In my experience, negative childhood experiences stem from our misinterpretations, miscommunications, and misunderstandings. Your age at the time of the negative event will determine the way you interpret it, and how deeply it lands. The tone and delivery of a negative message conveyed by a parent will determine how you accept it as your truth. The misunderstanding about yourself, as a result, is before you realize how very little it had to do with "you." Instead, it's how much it had to do with the emotional state of the parent you had the problem with.

This is something I tell every one of my clients before we begin our work together. Working on core issues for many of us will include itemizing negative events with our parents. They're our main people, the mirrors through which we learn to see ourselves very early on. They weren't given any handbooks on how to raise us. Given their background and their circumstances, they did the best they could at the time. We're not throwing stones at them, persecuting them, or playing the blame game. Not at all.

For your own sake, and for the sake of your health, you have to be absolutely ready to look at everything and leave no stone unturned. In your own life experiences everything is important and impactful, and everything counts and matters. When it comes to you finally learning how to play on the same team instead of against yourself, the past is worth a second look.

Emotional entitlement is a big part of owning the problem, and an important tenant of EFT. If there is resistance or denial, I always suggest that my client work on guilt before we even begin a session. If they are motivated, they will, and it accelerates our sessions with lightning speed.

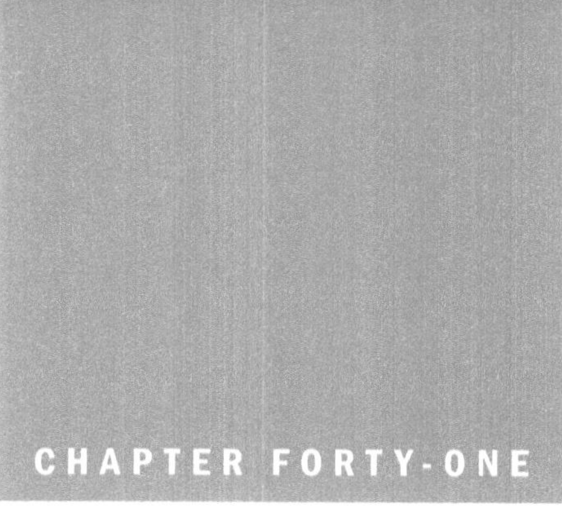

Now Your Turn

Before we even begin, my clients are required to take the time for themselves for quiet reflection and create their own Storyboard list. It's a list of issues to work through and keep our focus. If I see them intellectualizing themselves into a corner, that tells me they just aren't ready, and we start with current issues. Eventually, all roads lead backward, and they begin to recognize the importance of their past in their own time.

Parental issues are very big. In fact, they're huge and they are powerful, so the less negative events with them you hang onto, the happier and the healthier you'll be. Love is a healing energy, and once you relearn how to apply it to yourself and your life, it supports your own self-nurturing and self-respect.

Wonderful things happen when you learn to let go of old problems on a cellular level, energetically. Your natural born intuitive sense becomes fine tuned without all the clutter of negative background noise and doubts inside your head. Without a doubt, trusting your inner voice becomes second nature the way it was meant to be. Not only that, but when you clear the space of a negative memory, and you do enough of them, the positive, happier memories pop up and take their place! It happens naturally without you even trying! Think about it, you're finally working with yourself instead of against, playing on your own team, joyful thoughts instead of the negative thoughts are within your reach, and to top it all, the greatest upside is better health!

Many authors have described how writing their autobiography was dreadful, painful and cathartic. I've been very candid about my life, and I can tell you in all honesty that writing about my past was not dreadful or painful or sad. Not in the least. As for cathartic, that already happened through EFT. That's real-time testimony of how well this stuff works. It was also a good way for me to re-test for unresolved emotional remnants. My results were clean! Gone forever, thank you very much, and so can yours.

I have nothing but gratitude for what I've been through in my life. I've learned so much about myself and people along the way. Those lessons have been invaluable life experiences that I was able to break through, and gave me the confidence that I can help you too.

On our website, EFTOne.com, you can learn how to use EFT to overcome anything life throws your way. No matter what you've been through in your past, or what your current challenges are, there is hope. Even if this is the first time you've ever heard of EFT, things can and do get better. Millions of others, including myself, who've helped themselves are living proof.

> **"The mission of <u>EFTOne.com</u> is to help as many people as possible understand and use the elegant techniques of EFT to overcome health problems, improve their lives and protect themselves from the cumulative effects of negative stresses."**

This is my message and the purpose of our website: to restore your health and to improve and empower your life. EFT is life-changing, and it works. It means you have to be ready for the fast, permanent and positive changes that take place when you use it.

Helping people is what I was born to do. Using an amazing energy psychology technique like EFT to ease your mind and heal your body is what I consider my life's work. It's what I'm innately good at, it's what I do. I'm so grateful for this experience of sharing my life with you for the sole purpose of giving you hope.

Even I, the suspicious, practical thinking Midwestern doubter of the esoteric, changed my tune. I used it on myself and applied it to every aspect of my life. The domino effect of this deep self-work is that it allows personal growth. And that contributes to allowing yourself to catch up, and meet your full potential. It frees you up to reach your goals and dreams without the sabotage. It can and will turn your life into the reality you've always imagined. It's our birthright, from before the wounds of life began.

I'm the same girl who marched back into that airline VP's office and said, "This is who I am, and this is why you need me." This time around, I have the strength and the courage to be <u>her</u> all the time.

My personal power interview was a great example of the inner power we all possess even though once hired, I fell back into my usual way of seeing myself. It was a wonderful insight into the power of the real me. With EFT I was able to peel the layers, remove the baggage that had accumulated in my mind, my soul if you will, and become that person again. It was like a special 'gift' from a deep inner part of myself, showing me "here's who you really are, here's your real power."

If you've come this far in my book, this is who I am. This is why you need me; for whatever's not working in your life right now, and especially if you're sick, you simply have to try tapping, and I'll show you how. You will never know the extent of the power that your mind has over your body unless you learn how to access that ability. In our next book, Body Mind Renewal, I explain how to find the emotional trends of every illness, disease, and pain syndrome imaginable. I offer you information based on my real-time clinical experience and repetition of findings with literally thousands of seriously ill clients.

Unfortunately, by the time it occurs to them that there is an emotional part of the equation, many of my seriously ill clients have exhausted all other sources of help. But, because insurance doesn't cover "alternative" or "naturalistic" approaches to health and healing, they have already depleted their finances. Because of finances, they generally have a very tight 'session limit' (I can only do 6 sessions, etc.) and they want a miracle, ASAP. They want to undo a lifetime of negative emotional layering. Or, rather, they want ME to undo it for them.

And, on top of all that, they almost always are at a Stage 4 of their cancer or illness.

Wouldn't it be wonderful if they had learned about EFT sooner? Had started applying it right at the beginning of the illness. Or even better, had used it as prevention, as an ongoing 'de-stressing' of the mind's emotions, and their effect on the body.

My vision, my mission, is to help as many people as possible realize the beauty of having a self-help tool like EFT; to realize that ALL illness has an emotional component and that addressing it is just as important as all the drugs, diets, vitamins, minerals, herbs, needles, magnets, resonant frequencies and whatever else has been offered as a solution.

Although there are schools of thought and well-known charts correlating organ systems and emotions, my experiences have led me to understand a deeper complexity. It's never a simple formula of instructions. Or even the whole story. It's easy to fall into an over-simplification or over-generalization and miss the mark. FYI: internal organs (as well as the skin) carry more than one emotion. Just so you know.

My emotional healing wasn't from years of psychotherapy, positive thinking or positive affirmations. It was a head-on collision with the parts of my past that were negative -- using EFT to work through them methodically. In doing so, I cleared the way for my present, and ultimately, my future.

Once overlooked and distanced from us by modern medicine, energetic healing is finally being recycled back into current healthcare's conscious awareness. Thus far, I have never seen anything work as fast as simply thinking about a negative problem, and tapping on a few acupoints. It's of the utmost importance to connect the emotional dots and address the hidden layer of health, your emotional body.

The beauty of this technique is that it's a personalized tool to restore yourself. You do it yourself, anytime, anywhere, specifically for in-the-moment first aid. That in itself is amazing. But when you address those deeper core emotional layers that have stunted parts of your growth for years, there occurs a deep and profound healing of the heart. It's that new-found loving energy that creates homeostasis of the physical body.

All of it is accomplished just by releasing the worries and regrets of the mind. Imagine that?

Therein lies the power of EFT.

⟨❈⟩

The End

...or, the Beginning?

The Basics in a Nutshell

If you are totally new to the concept of EFT and tapping, or just want a quick bare-bones review, Appendix I is for you.

Appendix II explores the history of Energy Psychology and energy therapies in general.

Appendix III gives a quick history of the development of EFT.

Appendix IV is a rather large listing of links to research and academic articles on things related to EFT.

Appendix V has links to the all-important ACE Study.

OK, Newbies! There are two CRUCIAL points I want to make: master the Basic Formula AND really, really understand the concept of the Storyboard Procedure. With those two tools you can make powerful changes in your life, present and future.

The Basic Formula, as it's referred to, is the core process of EFT. For the sake of brevity I'm going to only present the Short Version of the Basic formula, leaving out the 9-Gamut procedure. It involves several things:

1. Selecting a SPECIFIC memory or event.
2. Assigning a number (0-10) reflecting the current intensity of the emotion(s) associated with the event or memory.
3. Coming up with a Reminder Phrase to keep you focused on the issue; the mind does tend to wander, you know?

4. Tapping with 2 or 3 fingers on the 'karate chop point' (see the illustration in the Introduction) while stating the problem or issue. The classic EFT phrasing is "even though I have this (problem), I deeply and completely love and accept myself." For example: Even though I have this fear of spiders, I deeply and completely love and accept myself."

5. Tapping on the 13 acupoint spots while repeating your Reminder Phrase. Example: "my fear of spiders." It is considered important to tap relatively firmly and to tap at least 7-10 times on each acupoint.

6. After tapping the points while repeating the Reminder Phrase (to keep focused on the ONE specific event/memory), stop and reevaluate the intensity of the memory on the 0-10 scale, then repeat the process until the intensity is a Zero. Each 'round' of the tapping process takes approximately 60 seconds.

The "Storyboard Procedure" starts with you coming up with a list, your very own "shit-list", as some would refer to it, of all the crap or emotional garbage that has happened to you over the course of your life...sometimes even before you were out of the womb, pre-natal stresses of your mom that energetically affected you. This list then becomes the focus of your tapping sessions with yourself, the goal being to bring everything on the list down to a zero intensity.

My shit-list turned out to be pages long, over four legal notepad pages, front and back. I listed traumatic events as far back as I could go; not only childhood memories, but the years of experiences accumulated afterward. They were all easy for me to remember; in fact, I knew them all by heart.

While some people report feeling shame and embarrassment because their list will be so long, I didn't give a hoot about how long my list of issues was. Who was going to see them anyway? I had a motive: I wanted to feel better inside.

I listed every single one of my childhood traumas, including my teens and young adulthood. I also included the ones I had forgotten about that popped up out of nowhere. I wanted them gone. So, diligently, every single day, I made it a point to knock off three negative events from my past. I did that for three years straight while I refined my EFT skills. I was working my way up the ladder to Master Practitioner.

Instead of feeling overwhelmed, embarrassed or damaged by the size of the list of my personal issues, I set aside my self-judgement, and worked on three issues per day, every day.

I thought about how each memory felt now, in the moment, and not how it felt back then, and wrote down the intensity level alongside each one from 0-10. Zero means there is no feeling, and 10 is you're either crying or ready to go ballistic.

The way EFT worked for me, (we all react a bit differently) was that it fragmented my visual memories so that I couldn't piece them back together in my mind's eye. And I couldn't get any kind of a charge out of them. I also learned that when I "yawned" after some tapping rounds, the intensity of the issue had either gone down dramatically or was gone completely.

In my years of working with the underlying emotions of serious diseases and pain syndromes, I discovered that there are a variety of ways for the body to express letting go. It used to scare me at first, but several thousand clients later, I know better. These are exaggerated, but temporary, physical reactions that can occur when your body is sick with an illness. This includes vomiting, sleepiness, shivering, shakiness, flatulence, diarrhea, or just having a really great bowel movement for the first time in a long time. It's still an energy release, and an indication that you've still accomplished something good because your body just spoke-up. You may not like what it's saying in the moment, but it's letting you know there is a movement of energy!

I have found over my years as a practitioner and workshop teacher that one of the most common failures in using EFT is to NOT take the time and energy necessary to create and work through a Storyboard Procedure. In fact, years ago I produced a series of videos called "The EFT Dropout Syndrome"[13] that explored the 3 most common reasons people stopped using EFT after a while; even those who were wildly excited about the possibilities. Guess what the #1 Reason was? Right. Failure to do a Storyboard list.

---

[13] To view the video on the #1 reason click here. https://www.youtube.com/watch?v=-OLAUwb4Zv8

So that's it. Learn the Basic Formula until it's second nature and DO the Storyboard Procedure. You can download a copy of my unique Storyboard Procedure template here: https://www.dropbox.com/s/5spczdh1vlnt09x/PPP the Template.pdf?dl=0

A few words on the power of EFT and the caution that should be exercised...use EFT responsibly, both on yourself and on other people. It is a wonderful set of tools for improving your life, but every human being is a unique, complex system of matter, energy and spirit and any intervention should be made with caution and according to common sense, giving proper consideration to the possible consequences. We strongly suggest that its application takes place within a larger program of therapy or personal development.

EFT can tempt you to use it for quickly fixing some problems, even serious and chronic ones, or to experiment with changes that could possibly have deep effects on the personality. It's the first time in human history that literally everybody (even a child!) can quickly learn and apply such a powerful method for changing emotions and thoughts. So, act responsibly and with caution, in order to enjoy the power of EFT with no serious negative side effects.

We cannot stress enough the fact that to use EFT professionally, on clients, it is absolutely necessary to get proper training in it and not rely solely on information from the Web and books. EFT can help you achieve incredible results in a very short time, if you get to know it well enough and practice it enough.

Unless you involve the help of an experienced EFT Practitioner, you should always follow common sense and not go places where you don't belong, that is, to attempt to treat with EFT cases outside your educational and work experience.

History of Energy Therapies

This is an abbreviated history of the concept of bioenergies, meridians, acupoints (tapping points), and acupuncture.

Energy Psychology (EP) is a group of healing techniques that manipulate subtle energies in the body. It does this while addressing mental or emotional components.

Energy, aka "Qi", "Chi," "Prana," etc. is derived from the foods and liquids we take in for nourishment and hydration. It's in the air we breathe, and all the other subtle elements that we absorb into our bodies. It is conceptualized as the vital life force.

We now know that the origins of ancient acupuncture and "meridians" predate ancient Chinese medicine's written record. And in fact are actually not an exclusive possession of the ancient Chinese at all. The knowledge spread to the four corners of the world and as it turns out, all the ancients knew a little something about this stuff.

Meridians are a network of channels that run over and through the body, conducting the flow of this vital energy, "Qi," through the body.

There are twelve "Organ Meridians" that are the same twelve meridians used in EFT "Tapping." This network of channels transports this energy to the related internal organs and body parts, including the surrounding tissues and blood vessels along its route.

Named for the related internal organ, the meridians are: Lung, Large Intestine, Stomach, Spleen, Heart, Small Intestine, Bladder, Kidney, Pericardium, Triple Warmer (adrenals), Gall Bladder, and Liver.

Acu-points are places along the meridians where this energy is accessible or close to the surface of the skin. Research studies have shown that the electrical conductivity of acu-points is 100X greater than that of the surrounding areas.

To stimulate an Acu-point, you can tap on them with your fingertips, apply pressure and rub with your fingertips, use acupuncture needles, or by moxibustion - burning an herb at the end of the acupuncture needle.

Sickness is a disorganization or "imbalance" of energy within the meridian, inside the organ, or more often than not, both.

The Papyrus Ebers of 1550 BC is the most important of ancient Egyptian medical texts. It refers to a book on the subject of certain "vessels" that correspond to the 12 organ meridians of acupuncture.

An isolated tribe in Brazil uses a more primitive form of acupuncture needles. They shoot tiny arrows with a blowpipe onto the body of the afflicted, using the same acu-points.

Indigenous people of Alaska, Canada, and Greenland practice acupuncture the original, primitive way: by using sharp stones as was first recorded by the ancient Chinese. This was before the development of needles.

Corresponding with the method of "Auricular" or ear acupuncture, the Bantu people of South Africa "scratch" the acu-points to cure disease. They would treat sciatica by cauterizing a part of the ear with a hot metal probe (ancient moxibustion).

More recently the 1991 discovery of the frozen, mummified body of a 5,300-year-old Chalcolithic (Copper Age) man. German hikers found the body at the border of the Austrian-Italian Tyrolean Alps. This discovery predates the first ancient Chinese acupuncture texts by 2000 years.

Called the "Iceman", he was a prehistoric European herdsman (deduced by his tools) who lived in mountainous isolation. It's important to note that this man was not Chinese, or from India. He was a European home-boy. He was about 30 years old when he was shot in the back with an arrow ending his life and turning him into a human popsicle on top of a glacier for 5,300 years. He never saw it coming.

Through DNA analysis, scientists found that he still has 19 genetic relatives living in Austria's Tyrol region today. That suggests his genes shopped locally and didn't cat around very far from home.

With his discovery we now had proof that more than one ancient culture - on more than one continent - had the knowledge of healing through the meridian energy pathways. Forensic scientists found 57 "therapeutic" (not "ornamental") tattoos made from fireplace soot on various parts of his body. These show an early type of acupuncture treatment. These simple tattoos are right on, or very near "modern" acupuncture points. Points used to treat chronic low back pain, joint pain, abdominal pain, and intestinal parasites.

In correlation with those tattooed "treatment spots" forensic scientists found that his stomach contents showed evidence of whipworms and bacteria related to ulcers. He also suffered from lactose intolerance, degenerative disc disease in his low back, and severe osteoarthritis in one knee and both ankles.

Thousands of years later, acupuncture, one of many healing techniques from the old wisdom, is still widely used today.

It's important to point out that acupuncture evolved to treat physical problems, not emotional problems. There are acupuncture practitioners today that will use it to relax a patient, or to relieve severe generalized anxiety. Yet, acupuncture does not have a systematic way of applying this method to emotional problems. Emotional Freedom Techniques (EFT) does. Simply stated, traditional acupuncture and acupressure are not viewed as psychological treatments.

"[It seems that] there is a coherent worldview...that emanates from many cultural and disciplinary perspectives, and that describes the world in energetic terms...Key tenets of this worldview include:

- the existence of a universal life force or vital energy flowing through and available to all beings;
- the existence of a subtle energy system or biofield that interpenetrates the physical anatomy of the human body and extends outward beyond it;

- the idea that in ill health, the human energetic field is out of balance or congested, free flow is blocked, which diminishes the normal self-healing capacity…"[14]

The term biofield describes "a field of energy and information, both putative and subtle, that regulates the homeodynamic function of living organisms and may play a substantial role in understanding and guiding health processes." "Evidence for the existence of the biofield now exists, and current theoretical foundations are now being developed."[15]

The term biofield fills the need for a unifying concept to bridge traditional and contemporary explanatory models of energy medicine and provides a common language for aspects of both clinical practice and scientific research that focus on energy fields of the body.

The following are links to academic articles throwing light on the history of Energy Psychology.

https://www.chi.is/wp-content/uploads/2017/04/1-CHI-Research-Editorial-Exploring-the-Biofield-CHI.pdf

https://www.chi.is/wp-content/uploads/2017/04/2-CHI-Research-Biofield-Science-and-Healing-An-Emerging-Frontier-in-Medicinepdf.pdf

https://www.chi.is/wp-content/uploads/2017/04/3-CHI-Research-Biofield-Science-and-Healing-History-Terminology-and-Concepts.pdf

https://www.chi.is/wp-content/uploads/2017/04/5-CHI-Research-Biofield-Science-Current-Physics-Perspectives.pdf

---

[14] . A consideration of the Perspectives of Healing Practitioners on research Into energy Healing Sara L. Warber, MD; Rtsalyn L. Bruyere, DD; Ken Weintrub, MA; Paul Dieppe MD, FRCP, FFPH

[15] . Biofield Science: Current Physics Perspectives Menas C. Kafatos, PhD; Gaétan Chevalier, PhD; Deepak Chopra, MD, FACP; John Hubacher, MA; Subhash Kak, PhD; Neil D. Theise, MD

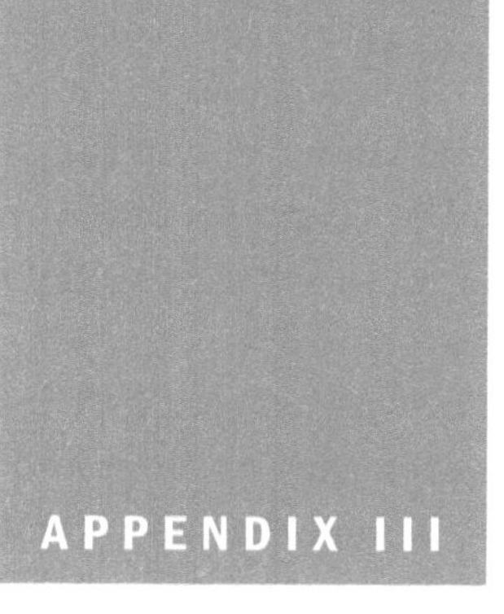

History of EFT

Frequently called "emotional acupuncture", EFT has its origins in the work of an American chiropractic physician, Dr. George Goodhart.

Back in 1964, after studying acupuncture and the correlations of the meridians, conventional neurology and visceralsomatic reflexes, Dr. Goodheart developed a procedure using muscle strength testing that allowed insights into the body's response to subtle energies, both positive and negative. He applied pressure with his fingertips rather than needles to stimulate the meridian points. He called the new method Applied Kinesiology.

Applied Kinesiology uses muscle testing to determine the appropriateness of any form of treatment. It acts to override conscious thought and speak to the body's subconscious mind. It's really quite cool, and if you know how to do it properly, as a physician, you learn a lot about a patient.

Much to their surprise, the patient learns a lot about themselves as well because the muscle response is beyond their conscious control. It's always a real eye-opener for them.

In the 1970's Australian psychiatrist Dr. John Diamond learned of Dr. Goodheart's work and created his own spin on Applied Kinesiology (AK), creating a variation of it by adding affirmations while the patient stimulated certain acupoints on their body. He found that it could bring about changes in emotional states as well as physical conditions. He called it "Behavioral Kinesiology."

In the early 1980's an American clinical psychologist, specializing in anxiety and phobias, Dr. Roger Callahan, was the first to combine tapping on the acupoint and modern psychology, calling it "Thought Field Therapy."

A client named Mary was his very first "one minute wonder" and the absolute game changer for his findings and his new technique.

Mary suffered from extreme fear of water. She couldn't be in same room with a pool, or in a backyard with a pool, it was that intense. The thought of taking a bath in a tub full of water, or being in a room with a full bathtub, was enough to put her into a full-blown panic attack. She hated the feeling of water on her skin in general. To put it mildly, Mary was an anti-aquatic mess!

Callahan worked with her for two years using cognitive behavioral therapy with no success. One day during a session Mary told him the sensation of fear she was having was located in her stomach. While she was talking about her fear of water he had her tap under her eyes, on a point on the stomach meridian.

Not only did she feel the fear release from her stomach, but she suddenly called out that she was no longer afraid of water!

Callahan's initial gut reaction was yeah, right, lady and chickens have lips too. He didn't take it seriously because it seemed highly unlikely. But she definitely had his attention when she sprang up from her chair, ran outside to the swimming pool, and began splashing water on her face! She'd never been able to get that close to a pool before. He remembered she couldn't swim so he ran out to the pool after her to make sure she didn't fall in. Her results were permanent. You heard me, yes, permanent!

Having a stunning success with Mary, Dr. Callahan explored tapping on specific meridian points to treat other types of phobias. Over time he developed tapping sequences for different emotional issues, sequences he called "Algorithms."

The appropriateness of these algorithms was determined for each client by muscle testing. However exciting the results, Callahan's "Thought Field Therapy" (aka "TFT") had its pitfalls. For one thing, it was far from a self-help technique. The process of working with the algorithms was long and tedious, and had to be administered by a therapist who was also expert in muscle testing for the most accurate results.

In the early 1990's Gary Craig, a highly successful personal performance coach and Stanford trained engineer, studied with Dr. Callahan to learn how to use TFT. It was his engineer's left brain that asked the question: why not tap on all twelve meridian points in one single algorithm and cover everything?

His discovery was that using one single algorithm not only worked, it was faster. And best of all, you could do it yourself without muscle testing. Distancing himself from Callahan's work, he called his technique "Emotional Freedom Techniques," EFT for short.

With profound insight Gary understood the importance, the impact this new self-help technique would have on the world.

As EFT practitioners back in the early years, we really were on the ground floor of this "healing high rise" as he would say. He wanted the world to know about it. His website, Emofree.com, went global with written testimonials from his practitioners that reached millions of people worldwide.

For many years he actually gave away his EFT how-to manual for free, no monetary gain on his part, it was a free download for anyone to learn it. Gary Craig was a standout philanthropist in the realm of self-help, nobody did that sort of thing back then without a profit. Because of his generosity, EFT is now the most influential and acknowledged method of Energy Psychology in the world.

After Gary retired in early 2010 and turned over the articles and testimonials from <u>Emofree.com</u> to Dr. Dawson Church (<u>EFTUniverse. com</u>), any number of websites sprang up with programs to teach and certify you in EFT; variety and spinoff was the flavor of the day. However, in my professional opinion the original uncomplicated version that Gary Craig developed is powerful and elegant and the basics easy to learn by anyone. I've included links in Appendix IV to those that I suggest you look at.

EFT Research and Links

As of 2018 the amount of research into the validity and effectiveness of EFT continues to grow.

1. Over 100 published studies using meridian tapping approaches
2. 50 random controlled studies
3. 98% Positive results
4. 4 Meta-Analyses for EFT
5. 5 Systematic reviews
6. Hundreds of Case Studies

Here's a link to a super quick overview of current research into EFT:
http://www.energypsych.org/resource/resmgr/research/Science_Behind_EP_Quick_Fact.pdf

ACEP's (Association for Comprehensive Energy Psychology) list of references on Energy Psychology; a very comprehensive list
https://www.energypsych.org/page/EPReferences.

ACEP's list of references on Energy Psychology research
https://www.energypsych.org/page/Research_Landing

A neuroscience look at three interlocking brain processes (amygdala deactivation, polyvagal theory and memory reconsolidation) that offer insights into why EFT is so effective in treating the effects of trauma.
https://acepblog.org/2014/10/30/energy-psychology-an-integrated-neuroscience-paradigm/

EFT Universe's lists of research.
https://eftuniverse.com/research-studies/eft-research

Association for Advancement of Meridian Energy Techniques.
https://aametinternational.org/discover-eft/eft-science-research/

Great article by D. Feinstein, PhD published in the American Psychological Associations journal.
http://www.innersource.net/ep/images/stories/downloads Acupoint_Stimulation_Research_Review.pdf

Research on comparison of EFT and Cognitive Behavioral Therapy
https://www.liebertpub.com/doi/pdf/10.1089/ACM.2015.0316

PTSD research with EFT
https://www.ncbi.nlm.nih.gov/pmc/articles/PMC5499602/

Kelly Brogan, MD, Wholistic Psychiatrist's article on epigenetic and beliefs.
https://kellybroganmd.com/gamechanging-science/

How stress affects cortisol levels which impact inflammatory responses and the immune systems.
https://medicalxpress.com/news/2012-04-stress-disease-reveals-inflammation-culprit.html

Stress, trauma and autoimmune diseases
http://www.greenmedinfo.com/blog/stress-trauma-and-auto immune-disease-it-s-not-all-your-head

Very good article by David Feinstein, PhD
http://www.innersource.net/ep/images/stories/downloads/Acupoint_Stimulation_Research_Review.pdf.

Research article on the effects of EFT on stress biochemistry.
https://journals.lww.com/jonmd/Abstract/2012/10000/The_Effect_of_Emotional_Freedom_Techniques_on.12.aspx

Research into biophotons and meridian paths.
https://www.liebertpub.com/doi/abs/10.1089%2Facm.2005.11.171.

Research on the Primo vascular system and meridians.
https://www.jams-kpi.com/article/S2005-2901(13)00208-2/abstract

Powerpoint presentation on the Primo Vascular systems and its relation to the meridian system.
https://www.slideshare.net/thorntonstreeter/primo-vascular-meridian-system-2016?qid=d7e7cdd8-de3f-437b-832c-0cde9f9f52ea&v=&b=&from_search=7

Anther article on acupuncture meridians.
https://www.healthcmi.com/Acupuncture-Continuing-Education-News/1230-new-ct-scans-reveal-acupuncture-points

EFT and brain scans research.
https://bond.edu.au/intl/news/49213/world-first-brain-scan-research-shows-tapping-effective-combating-food-cravings

Another listing of research.
http://www.tappingsolutionfoundation.org/science-and-research/

Article on link between trauma and physical illness.
https://wakeup-world.com/2017/07/25/the-unmistakable-link-between-unhealed-trauma-and-physical-illness/

The ACE Study

ACE study questionnaire
https://www.evernote.com/l/AJCbgrPVrEtKVI152mn28rXUMz
CUVIj7nJM

Vincent J. Felitti, MD article on ACE and Adult Health: Turning
gold into lead
https://www.evernote.com/l/AJAtYSjn1u5AkqC7OKNWAUlaV
WW0o6kF8II

The ACE Quiz from NPR
https://www.npr.org/sections/health-shots/2015/03/02/3870
07941/take-the-ace-quiz-and-learn-what-it-does-and-doesnt-mean

CDC link to ACE study
https://www.cdc.gov/violenceprevention/acestudy/index.html

ACE report on Chronic Disease & Childhood Trauma
https://www.evernote.com/l/AJBd34xnLMVOh6NJhUqo6ClAn
OxRVB0pjOY

Dr. Rossanna M. Massey

Biological embedding of childhood adversity: from physiological mechanisms to clinical implications

https://bmcmedicine.biomedcentral.com/articles/10.1186/s12916-017-0895-4

www.ingramcontent.com/pod-product-compliance
Lightning Source LLC
Chambersburg PA
CBHW031107250726
48655CB00004B/1618